MEDICAL ETHICS

MEDICAL ETHICS
PRINCIPLES, PERSONS, AND PROBLEMS

JOHN M. FRAME

Distributed by
BAKER BOOK HOUSE
Grand Rapids, Michigan

Manufactured in the United States of America.
Typesetting by Thoburn Press, Tyler, Texas.

Library of Congress Cataloging-in-Publication Data

Frame, John M., 1939-
    Medical ethics : principles, persons, and problems / John M. Frame
       p.   cm.
    Bibliography: p.
    Includes indexes.
    ISBN 0-87552-261-0 :
    1. Medical ethics. 2. Medicine—Religious aspects—Christianity.
  3. Evangelicalism.   I. Title.
    [DNLM: 1. Ethics, Medical. 2. Religion and Medicine.
  BL 65.M4 F813m]
  R725.56.F73 1989
  174'.2—dc19
  DNLM/DLC
  for Library of Congress   88-29050
                                               CIP

92   91   90   89   88   5   4   3   2   1

CONTENTS

ANALYTICAL OUTLINE

PREFACE

For some years I have been working on a book called *Doctrine of the Christian Life* (hence *DCL*), which I hope eventually to publish in my *Theology of Lordship* series as one of the sequels to my recently published *Doctrine of the Knowledge of God* (hence *DKG*).[1] *DCL* now exists in the form of a 250-page lecture outline. It presents in some detail my general approach to ethics, some critiques of alternative ethical philosophies and theologies, and a survey of some ethical problems presented as applications of the Ten Commandments.

The book you are now reading is not *DCL*. The present volume came about when Dr. Jay Adams asked me to lecture on medical ethics to two conferences of Christian counsellors. I felt that the somewhat elementary material in *DCL* was not challenging enough for these conferences, so I tried to develop something a little deeper,

1. Phillipsburg, N.J.: Presbyterian and Reformed Publishing Co., 1987.

something that would address the hard issues with which these counsellors were wrestling.

In this volume, therefore, I have not said much about basic epistemology; that is covered in *DCL* and in *DKG*. (Those interested in learning more about my "three perspectives" should get the latter book.) Nor does this volume include much discussion of ethical theories other than my own. At the counselling conference I was able to assume a broad base of common ground on these matters, and so readers of this book will have to tolerate my starting points.

I expect many to disagree with the positions taken in this volume. Controversy always accompanies discussions of difficult questions. I don't expect this book to settle anything once and for all. Much of my own thinking in these areas is tentative, perhaps more tentative than the language of the book itself may suggest. I do hope that the book will encourage discussion of these matters among its readers, discussion that may in time lead to more substantial answers than those advanced here.

I wish to acknowledge indebtedness, first, to those whom I cited in *DKG*, who continue to have great influence on my thought and my formulations. (John Hughes, who edited and typeset *DKG* to near perfection, is editing this volume as well, and for that I am very grateful.) Beyond those, I wish to acknowledge the special help of Dr. Franklin E. Payne, Dr. Hilton Terrell, and the Rev. James B. Jordan, all of whom read a previous version of this book and made a great many valuable suggestions. Although I have often followed their suggestions, sometimes I have not, and the blame for all the inadequacies of this book is mine alone. Thanks also to Jay Adams, whose role in the production of this book I mentioned earlier. Jay has been so wonderfully encouraging that it has always been difficult for me to say No to him. Had anyone else asked me to lecture to those counsellors, this book would probably never have been written. Thanks, too, to my dear wife and the children for helping me maintain perspective, and, above all, to the Lord Jesus, "who loved me and gave himself for me" (Gal. 2:20).

INTRODUCTION

This book deals with some of the more difficult questions in the field of medical ethics and with the methods that are available to evangelical Christians to resolve those questions.

Over the last fifteen years, Evangelicals have developed a consensus that abortion is wrong, except possibly if and when it is needed to save the life of a mother. How have we come to that moral conclusion? Well, Evangelicals do use some of the same arguments that Roman Catholics, pro-life Jews, and secularists employ: the unborn child is genetically unique and thus not part of his mother's body; sonograms reveal that even the youngest fetuses subject to abortion are capable of purposive movement and terrible pain.[1] But for Evangelicals, whether they admit it or not in this

---

1. The latter fact has been documented, for example, by Dr. Bernard Nathanson for the film *The Silent Scream*.

1

context, the final argument against abortion is scriptural and exegetical, however indirect the bearing of the biblical texts. *Sola scriptura*: Scripture alone is the ultimate authority for human faith and
life. Scripture says it, we believe it, and that settles it.

Because of its commitment to *sola scriptura*, the methodological
clarity of evangelical ethics[2] seems to give it a tremendous advantage
over other ethical systems. Whatever else may be said about evangelical ethics, it seems that Evangelicals have a clear idea of how to
reach moral conclusions. In many cases, such as abortion, suicide,
and active-involuntary euthanasia,[3] for example, that is true; but
in other cases, Evangelicals have lacked that sort of clarity.

How, for example, should an Evangelical deal with the following
situation? The book *Health and Human Values*[4] begins with the story
of Joseph Saikewicz, a man of sixty-seven with a mental age of two
years, eight months, who has incurable, terminal leukemia. The
authors ask, Should his doctors put him through the terribly painful
treatments required to extend his life for a year or so when he lacks
the ability to understand the purpose of those treatments, or should
the doctors decline to treat him, offering him as much comfort as
possible? Evangelicals—especially those in the Reformed tradition—
might be inclined to cite the sixth commandment ("You shall not
murder") and its exposition in the Westminster Catechisms, which
interpret it to require the *preservation* of life, as a command to supply
to Mr. Saikewicz the medical treatment that can extend his life. But
do we not also invoke the sixth commandment to justify giving relief
to those who suffer and to justify minimizing their pain? If we truly
reverence human life, can we justify imposing terribly painful treatments on Mr. Saikewicz without his understanding and consent?

2. Although confessionally I adhere to the Reformed theological tradition, in
this book I refer to my position as "evangelical" because I am not focusing (explicitly!) on Reformed distinctives but on the commitment to scriptural authority that
unites all Evangelicals. In that respect, the Reformed tradition is part of the evangelical heritage.
3. "Active-involuntary euthanasia" refers to a type of so-called mercy killing in
which the victim is an involuntary participant and actions (in whose absence the
victim would not die) are taken by other parties to ensure his death, for example,
death by lethal injection.
4. F. Harron, M. D. Burnside, and T. Beauchamp (New Haven: Yale University
Press, 1984).

In such cases evangelical ethics lacks the methodological clarity we normally expect it to have, and evangelical ethicists often seem as bewildered as their liberal and secular counterparts. More frequently, evangelical ethicists ignore the methodologically unclear problems and prefer to discuss issues where the biblical data are more explicit or at least easier to work with. Franklin Payne's recent *Biblical/Medical Ethics* (Milford, Mich.: Mott Media, 1985) is a case in point. The book is excellent in many ways. Payne is strongly committed to biblical authority and discusses important matters that other texts omit. But Payne's discussion of "guidelines for casuistry" in cases of terminal illness is only three pages long (pp. 207-09), and it amounts to a declaration—unsupported by any biblical references—that currently common practices in such cases are acceptable. Payne does not wrestle at all with the most difficult types of problems. I'm not saying that Payne should have wrestled with these issues; his book is well worth the price, even without adequate "guidelines for casuistry."[5] But I am saying that someone should grapple with the unclear ethical issues and that Evangelicals have some unique resources for doing so. God's people genuinely need a biblically developed set of "guidelines for casuistry" in these "problem areas."

Generally speaking, recent books and articles on ethics are of two basic types. The first type focuses on Scripture and seeks to set forth its teachings on ethical questions. Authors whose writings fall into this category include Payne, John Jefferson Davis, Walter Kaiser, and Rousas Rushdoony and the other theonomists. The second type focuses on the "problem areas," on the kinds of issues raised by cases like Mr. Saikewicz's, where the answers are not cut-and-dried. Authors whose writings fall into this category include Tom Beauchamp, James Childress, James Gustafson, Joseph Fletcher, Joel Feinberg, Robert Veatch, and others.[6] Generally speaking, books of the first type are written by Evangelicals, and books of

---

5. Payne is currently working on two more books that will deal with harder cases.
6. The bibliography at the end of this book lists some representative works of these authors.

the second type are written by liberals and secularists.[7] Books of
the first type are usually better for the soul. We grow in holiness by
exposing ourselves to the teachings of the Word of God. Books of
the second type, however, help us to see how richly complicated
real-life ethical decision making is. Why, then, shouldn't there also
be a book that focuses on the "problem areas" from a self-consciously
evangelical point of view and that seeks to discern how the Word
of God applies to these issues? This is the sort of need that the present book seeks to address.

I do not believe that there are easy answers in these areas. Belief
in biblical authority does not, as we shall see, make everything
simple. I do believe, however, that having an absolute ethical standard makes a difference in the way we deliberate and that it will, at
times (though not always), lead us to different conclusions from
those who deny that standard. I also believe that an evangelical
commitment enables us to specify clearly where and why problems
arise and what methods will be most effective in helping us make
decisions. These are the issues upon which this book will focus.

As a general principle, I begin (as all Evangelicals must) by
reiterating *sola scriptura*: Scripture alone is our ultimate authority.
An ethical decision, however, involves more than knowledge of
Scripture. In a counselling session, for example, there are three
types of questions to be discussed:

1. What is your problem? What kind of situation have you
   gotten into?

2. What does God's Word say about it?

3. Are you the sort of person who in this situation is capable
   of doing what Scripture tells you to do? Are you regener-
   ate? If so, are you sufficiently mature in the faith?

Note three foci: the situation, the Word, the person.

7. When Evangelicals write the second type of book or article, they often don't
sound like Evangelicals. Either they don't draw on Scripture at all, or they draw
only on Scripture's broadest principles, such as love, justice, and human dignity,
which they leave relatively undefined from an exegetical perspective. One recent
example of that type of work is Lewis Smedes, *Mere Morality* (Grand Rapids: Wm.
B. Eerdmans Publishing Co., 1983), which despite its limited exegetical base contains a great deal of ethical wisdom.

Those three perspectives are, of course, interrelated. You cannot adequately understand yourself or your situation without a biblical perspective. Nor can you adequately understand the Word of God or your situation without understanding yourself as a sinner saved by grace.[8] Nor can you understand yourself or God's Word unless you can relate them practically to your situation.[9] A proper analysis of the situation, therefore, will include reference to Scripture and the self as vital aspects of the situation. A proper analysis of the self will include Scripture and the situation as the self's proper context. And a proper analysis of Scripture will include the applications of Scripture to the relevant situations and moral agents.[10]

Therefore studying Scripture, studying the situation, and studying the person are not three separate studies, that is, three studies with distinct subject matters. Rather, they are the same activity carried out with different emphases or foci. When we study Scripture, we focus on Scripture and we relate it to the situation and the self. I call this study the "normative" perspective. Similarly, focusing on the situation can be called the "situational" perspective, and focusing on the personal moral agent can be termed the "existential" perspective.

I believe that non-Christian ethics has uniformly tried to separate those three perspectives. Joseph Fletcher's "situational ethics" attempted to gain ethical direction by analyzing situations and persons in terms of "love," rather than in terms of any norms or "rules." Fletcher's principle of love, however, failed to provide ethical direction, and so Fletcher advocated rules of his own devising. Immanuel Kant tried to deduce an ethic from the dictates of the moral law considered apart from the situation in which decisions must be made, and Jean Paul Sartre sought to develop an ethic that considers only the decision maker and his "authenticity." Almost all contemporary ethical thinkers see these attempts as failures. But

8. Cf., for example, the first pages of Calvin's *Institutes*.
9. Relations among Scripture, situation, and self are explored in more detail in my *Doctrine of the Knowledge of God* (Phillipsburg, N.J.: Presbyterian and Reformed Publishing Co., 1987).
10. For example, you cannot tell what Scripture says about abortion unless you know what an abortion is. So, paradoxically, our knowledge of Scripture, that is, of its applications, presupposes knowledge of other things.

what we should remember is that the problems in non-Christian philosophies arise *because* of unbelief. Non-Christians are unable to keep the three perspectives together because they have no sovereign God who guarantees the coherence of His Word with His creation and with the needs of persons made in His image. Therefore our triperspectival ethical model is a distinctively Christian, indeed distinctively evangelical, ethical approach.

In the remainder of this book we will examine some of the relevant issues that are related to each of the three perspectives: the normative, the existential, and the situational. Under the normative perspective, I will discuss the unity of our obligation in the light of its various levels, aspects, and forms. Under the existential perspective, I will focus on the person-as-patient and his needs, rights, and responsibilities. And under the situational perspective, I will discuss some of the traditional problem areas for medical ethics.

1

THE NORMATIVE PERSPECTIVE:
FINDING GOD'S WILL

The Christian's norm—his necessary, authoritative, sufficient, and clear standard—is the Bible, the Scriptures of the Old and New Testaments. As we have seen, Scripture *functions* normatively as it is applied to situations and to persons. Although it is simple enough to define the Bible as the Christian's ethical norm, doing so raises many questions from several different disciplines. There are, of course, all the questions raised by modern biblical criticism and by modern science. And lying behind those two disciplines are the questions raised by modern philosophy. Rather than deal with those questions, however, in this book we will focus on those issues that are problems within evangelical ethics, that is, among ethicists who are already committed to Scripture as their norm.

A. THE QUESTION OF CONFLICT

First we must ask if there are any "conflicts of duty" (sometimes called "tragic moral choices") within a truly biblical ethic. One of the most common illustrations of such a possible conflict is the case of the Dutch family in World War II who were hiding Jews in their basement. The Nazis came to the door and asked if the family was hiding Jews. Should the family have said No and lied, or should they have said Yes and delivered the Jews to terrible, unjust deaths? The idea of a "conflict of duty" is that in this fallen world we sometimes find ourselves in situations where we cannot help doing wrong. We must disobey one divine command or another. Sin is, as it were, forced upon us by the situation.

Most ethicists take it as axiomatic that there are such conflicts. That's understandable among liberals and secularists; they believe that all moral rules have exceptions, because all rules are human rules. They do not believe that any rules are divinely revealed. Somewhat surprisingly, however, some Evangelicals also endorse this notion. For example, John Warwick Montgomery says:

> The Christian morality fully realizes the difficulty of moral decision and frequently a Christian finds himself in a position where it is necessary to make a decision where moral principle must be violated in favor of other moral principles, but he never vindicates himself in this situation. He decides in terms of the lesser of evils or the greater of goods, and this drives him to the Cross to ask forgiveness for the human situation in which this kind of complication and ambiguity exists.[1]

Montgomery says that we must sometimes violate moral principle—that is, God's law—because of the "human situation" in which we find ourselves. Although in such a situation we have no choice other than to sin, we must still ask God's forgiveness for that sin. In other words, the situation has forced us to sin against God: obeying one law of God has forced us to disobey another.

Similarly, Franklin Payne, to whom I referred earlier, quotes Kaye and Wenham (another evangelical source) with approval:

---

1. Montgomery, *The Suicide of Christian Theology* (Minneapolis: Bethany Fellowship, 1970), 69.

... we shall insist that evil remain evil even when, being the lesser evil, it appears the right thing to do; we shall do it with a heavy heart, and seek God's cleansing of our conscience for having done it.[2]

According to Kaye and Wenham, it is sometimes right to do evil, right to disobey God. But even though it is right, we must nevertheless ask forgiveness for it. Apparently in this case doing right is sinful. In my view that approach is unbiblical for the following reasons.

1. In Scripture it is never right to disobey a command of God, and it is never sinful to do right. The position of Kaye, Wenham, and Montgomery on this point is ethically confused at a basic level.

2. According to this view, the Scriptures, our fundamental ethical standard, would be contradictory; they would be telling us to do two incompatible things.[3]

3. Consider the christological implication of this view. Did Jesus face "conflicts of duties"? If so, then He too was guilty of sin; He too ought to have asked God's forgiveness, as the above authors demand. But if Jesus did *not* face such conflicts, then how can we say with the author of Hebrews that He "was tempted in every way, just as we are, yet was without sin" (4:15)? Either alternative is unacceptable, so the premise must be wrong. There are no "tragic moral choices."

4. And 1 Corinthians 10:13 promises that Christians need never fall into sin, a promise that is incompatible with the view under discussion.

There are, therefore, no "conflicts of duty," no "tragic moral choices." That would seem to make our ethical task fairly easy. But alas, that is not so. Many ethical cases are genuinely difficult, as the preceding example about the Dutch couple in World War II il-

2. Franklin Payne, *Biblical/Medical Ethics* (Milford, Mich.: Mott Media, 1985), 68; cf. 59. He quotes Bruce Kaye and Gordon Wenham, *Law, Morality and the Bible* (Downers Grove, Ill.: Inter-Varsity Press, 1978), 152-53. In correspondence, Payne has told me that he no longer holds this view.

3. In my *Doctrine of the Knowledge of God* I argue that the applications of Scripture constitute its meaning. Therefore if the applications are contradictory, then Scripture itself is contradictory. God gives us Scripture to direct our lives. Its authority entails that such direction will not confuse us by pointing in two opposite directions.

lustrates.[4] Why? There are several reasons. Sometimes we don't understand Scripture adequately. Sometimes we have an inadequate understanding of the situation to which Scripture is to be applied. And sometimes our own spiritual immaturity obscures matters in our minds and hearts. Again we should note the normative-situational-existential triad. I cannot account for all the sources of ethical difficulty, but I shall note some of them under each of those three categories.

B. LEVELS OF PRIORITY WITHIN SCRIPTURE

First, we need a better understanding of the nature of our norm, the Bible, and of how it governs us ethically. We need to be particularly aware that biblical principles are part of a *system* of divine law. As is typical in legal systems, not all principles are on the same level; some have "priority" over others. Differences in priority are one source of complication in ethical discussions, as the following points demonstrate.

1. Certain principles are more important than others: "I desire mercy and not sacrifice" (Matt. 9:13); "Leave your gift at the altar and be reconciled to your brother" (Matt. 5:24); "The weightier matters of the law" (Matt. 23:23).

2. Scripture assumes that in emergencies normal regulations may be transcended in the interest of human health and safety (cf., e.g., Matt. 12:4).

3. Lower authorities may (and must!) be disobeyed when they conflict with higher ones (Acts 5:29; Exod. 1:15-22; etc.). It is not, to be sure, always clear which authority is higher than which. God's authority is always supreme, and any authority that contra-

4. Often, believing in an authoritative, and therefore consistent, Bible makes ethical decision making even more difficult. For if the Bible is that kind of book, then we must find a *consistent* answer to our ethical questions, what 1 Corinthians 10:13 calls a "way to escape." We cannot be satisfied with a paradoxical-contradictory "tragic choice." Those who believe in tragic moral choice sometimes charge their opponents with seeking "easy answers." Actually, however, the shoe is on the other foot. Christians who do *not* believe in "tragic moral choice" often must struggle longer to find biblical solutions to tough ethical questions than those who believe in "tragic moral choice."

dicts God's Word must be disobeyed. But at lower levels, questions often arise. Calvin, for example, argued that "lesser magistrates" sometimes may or must resist tyrannical or unjust actions of the "higher magistrates," even though in most situations the lower authorities are to be subject to the higher (Rom. 13:1; 1 Pet. 2:13f.). That implies that such resistance, where justifiable, should be seen as obedience to a law higher than the tyrant, such as the basic constitution of the state (written or unwritten) or the law of God Himself.

4. Many biblical commands cannot be carried out instantaneously; some must wait on others. For example, I cannot study the Bible and evangelize my neighborhood simultaneously. We must therefore use our own God-given wisdom to determine how our time should be divided among the various divine mandates.

5. Many biblical commands are given to the whole church, not to individuals as such. Adam and Eve as individuals could not have replenished and subdued the earth (Gen. 1:28ff.). The apostles as individuals could not have taught "all nations" (Matt. 28:19). Individuals must each make some *contribution* toward these goals, but such contributions will vary greatly according to individual opportunities and gifts (see Rom. 12; 1 Cor. 12).

6. God is free to declare exceptions (or clarifications?) of various other sorts to the general principles of the law. "You shall not murder" allows for capital punishment (Gen. 9:6; Exod. 21:12), self-defense (Exod. 22:2), and lawful war (Deut. 20).

7. Developments in redemptive history bring about changes in human obligation. The completeness of Christ's sacrifice, for example, brought animal sacrifices to an end. The controversy over "theonomy"[5] largely deals with the question of to what extent other such changes have taken place.

8. Cultural changes also bring about modifications in the way biblical laws are applied in specific cases. Deuteronomy 22:8 commands the Israelites to fence in their roofs for safety's sake. Although that command is not relevant in a society where roofs

5. See Greg L. Bahnsen, *Theonomy in Christian Ethics* (Phillipsburg, N.J.: Presbyterian and Reformed Publishing Co., 1977, 1984). Bahnsen argues that the civil penalties of the Mosaic Law, such as stoning for adultery, are binding upon present-day civil governments. For a contrary view, see Meredith G. Kline, "Comments on an Old-New Error," *Westminster Theological Journal* 41 (1979): 172-89.

are not used for social activities, the general principle of protecting one's family and visitors still applies. And note that this is an example where the normative and situational perspectives overlap: a change in the situation brings about a change in the application of the norm.

9. Scripture evaluates moral actions, thoughts, and attitudes in four ways: in terms of prohibition, permission, commandment, and praise. These, too, can be described as four "levels" of obligation.

a. *Prohibition* is perhaps the easiest of these to deal with. God tells us "Don't," and we don't. This is, in a sense, the simplest form of moral instruction. Children understand "No" before they understand the more positive forms of moral instruction. The Ten Commandments are mostly written in a negative form that contributes to their intelligibility as the most fundamental stratum of the law and to their appropriateness for the Old Covenant, which was a time of spiritual immaturity.

In medical ethics the fundamental negative principle is the sixth commandment, "You shall not murder." The general principle of respect for human life also forbids any kind of physical harm (Exod. 22:12-36). God even forbids His people to put others in *danger* of such harm. (I believe that this is part of what God had in mind by legislating "cities of refuge" in the Old Testament [Num. 35:22-28; Deut. 19:4ff.].) Accidental killing is a crime, because we ought to be supremely careful with human life. This is the background of Jesus' teaching that even anger and failing to be reconciled are forbidden (Matt. 5:21-24), for they are the roots of murder.

The moral obligation to be supremely careful with human life and not to take it accidentally is the fundamental principle of medical ethics: *primum non nocere*—"first, do no harm."[6] Those who administer medical treatment must seek to avoid even the *risk* of harm. In my opinion, this principle alone is adequate to rule out abortion except when and if an abortion is necessary to save a mother's life. Why? Because even if there is doubt about the personhood of the fetus, there is certainly a very high probability of

6. Called "nonmaleficence" in the useful discussion of Tom L. Beauchamp and James F. Childress, *Principles of Biomedical Ethics* (New York: Oxford University Press, 1979), 97ff.

such personhood, so that abortion always runs a high *risk* of destroying a human being. Although that is a simple principle, it is not one that is always easy to apply. Consider again the case of Joseph Saikewicz: On the whole, would chemotherapy be helpful or harmful to him? Defining what constitutes "harm" or "help" is not always easy. It involves making value-judgments and going through a process of "weighing" the evidence. Belief in biblical authority does not exempt us from that. Making value-judgments and weighing what constitutes "harm" and what constitutes "help" are the points at which many of the traditional problems of medical ethics arise.

b. *Permission* is the second type of evaluation that is sometimes explicit in Scripture, such as the permission to eat plants and meat (Gen. 1:29f.; 9:2f.). Usually, however, what Scripture permits is inexplicit. Generally speaking, permission includes everything that Scripture does not forbid. Therefore the scope of what Scripture permits is enormous and includes buying cabbage for dinner, wearing blue socks, taking a university degree in physics, and so forth. Theologians sometimes describe such things as *"adiaphora,"* "things indifferent," but I think that language is misleading. No act is indifferent in the sense of being morally neutral or in the sense of being irrelevant to our Christian walk. Everything we do is either good or bad, either right or wrong, either glorifying to God or not (1 Cor. 10:31; Rom. 14:23).

Certainly, then, all actions that are permitted by Scripture are to be evaluated by Scripture, not by our autonomous judgment. But since many actions are not mentioned explicitly in Scripture, we must have recourse to a broader, more general set of biblical principles. Generally speaking, eating meat is good; but when it makes a brother stumble, it is necessary to abstain (Rom. 14:20). Attending a football game is generally good, but not if it manifests idleness or Sabbath-breaking.

This sort of reasoning can be subtle and difficult, and of course it illustrates our need to understand situations if we are to apply Scripture properly. Use of a respirator may be good in one situation, bad in another. To agonize over the differences between situations is *not* necessarily a symptom of situational ethics; it may be part of our solemn responsibility before God's authoritative Word.

c. *Commands* are the third type of evaluation found in Scripture. Although many biblical commands are formulated negatively, the most central, the command to love, is emphatically positive, as are the fourth and fifth commandments, the cultural mandate (Gen. 1:28ff.), and the Great Commission (Matt. 28:19f.). The biblical ethic is not one of merely avoiding evil; it is one of pursuing good. Therefore we speak of the "principle of beneficence":[7] we have a duty to help those in need, just as the Good Samaritan helped the man who was injured on the road (also see Gal. 6:10).

Because of the principle of beneficence, it is always wrong to urge passivity out of respect for divine sovereignty. Occasionally Christians will challenge the use of a controversial treatment by saying that we should leave the matter in God's hands, as if by trying to help the patient by using the controversial treatment we are attempting to "play God." On the one hand, if a treatment is ethically wrong, the argument is legitimate. No one is so sick that we may transgress God's norms in order to heal. If we do, we *are* usurping God's prerogatives. On the other hand, if a treatment is not unethical, it is wrong to restrict its use simply because it involves human initiative and effort. Scripture tells us that God works through humans to save souls, and so, too, He works through humans to heal bodies. If it is not true that God works through human efforts, then *no* healing efforts can ever be justified, nor, for that matter, can human efforts in any other sphere of life. But because men and women have been created in God's image as His ministers on earth, there is indeed a sense in which we have been divinely appointed to "play God" in the healing of our neighbors.

Of course, God can heal when and where He chooses, miraculously or providentially. But such possibilities, however much we may pray for them, ought not to temper our zeal to provide medical help to those in need. God's ultimate intentions are secret, and Scripture warns us against governing our lives by speculating about God's secret will (Deut. 29:29). His *revealed* will is our guide (Matt. 4:7), and it tells us to help others.

That raises some problems. Obviously it is not possible for you or for me to help everyone in this world who needs help. If we

7. Ibid., 135ff.

tried, we would have no time for anything else, and we would still be unsuccessful. We must remember that even Jesus and the apostles, who were able to heal supernaturally, did not heal everyone who needed healing. How, then, can we be responsible, in some *general* way, to help other people? We need to remember what we said earlier about "levels" of obligations in Scripture, especially 5, where we noted that many biblical commands are given to the whole church, not to individuals. Individuals are to make a *contribution* to the healing of others, but various factors will determine what role each individual plays.

Some of these factors include the following.

(A) One's gifts and training. I am not competent to find a cure for cancer, but others may be.

(B) One's time and resources.

(C) A reasonable hope of success.

(D) Proximity. This seems to play a role in the Good Samaritan story and in the supernatural healings in Scripture. The Samaritan helped someone who was near him; proximity establishes a natural priority for beneficence. Ordinarily I have a greater duty to those in my vicinity than to those many miles away, though that is not to say that we have no obligation to those who are starving in Africa, for example. But because proximity establishes a natural priority for beneficence, ordinarily it would be wrong to turn away a sick stranger to give more money to those who are starving in Africa.

(E) Family relationships. There is a special biblical emphasis, buttressed by some of the strongest language in Scripture (1 Tim. 5:8), on meeting the needs of one's own family. The family's needs are the most "proximate" in terms of *(D)* above. Storing up an inheritance to leave to one's children is a good thing in Scripture and is not to be foregone in the interest of equalizing the distribution of one's wealth.

(F) Common faith. Note the order of priority in Galatians 6:10. The point is not that the needs of unbelievers are to be ignored (the text teaches the contrary) but that there is a kind of natural "proximity" among fellow believers that ought not to be ignored. If nothing else, we know (or ought to know) one another's needs better than we know the needs of unbelievers.

(G) Other responsibilities. The help we owe those in need is limited by the other responsibilities God has placed on us. For example, we owe God a tithe of our income, and we owe our employers an honest day's work. These responsibilities will sometimes limit our involvement in helping others. Furthermore, we have a right to a certain amount of rest, recreation, and nourishment.

(H) It is not wrong to love ourselves (Matt. 22:39). The sixth commandment covers suicide and requires us to maintain our own health. But loving ourselves in Scripture often must take second place to loving others. Thus self-sacrifice is legitimate. We are not always obligated to take the course most conducive to our own health and safety (John 15:13; Rom. 5:7f.; 2 Cor. 4:7-18; chaps. 11-12; Phil. 1:22-26; Heb. 11; 1 John 3:16).

Thus the relationship between nonmaleficence and benevolence is asymmetrical. Nonmaleficence is an absolutely universal principle because it describes our stance toward every other human being: we must never harm anyone.[8] Beneficence, however, is invariably selective. We cannot be beneficent to everyone all the time, not even to ourselves. We must be wise in the use of our time and energy, and we must not feel guilty every time we must attend to something other than works of mercy.

I am uneasy with this approach, however, because I do not wish to encourage a calculating spirit. Surely it would be wrong, when we see someone bleeding on the road, to carry out an elaborate cost/benefit/responsibility analysis before deciding to help. That would be the equivalent of asking, "Who is my neighbor?"—the question Jesus commends the Good Samaritan for not asking (see Luke 10:29ff.). And Paul testifies that he voluntarily renounced his "rights" for the sake of the church (1 Cor. 9; also see the references to self-sacrifice under (H) above). This attitude certainly goes beyond the principle that for X to have a duty toward Y "the benefit that Y will gain outweighs any harms that X is likely to suffer and does not present more than minimal risk to X."[9] Or would these exhortations more properly be discussed under the next heading?

8. Except, I would say, in cases where I believe that we are divinely authorized to do so, such as capital punishment and just warfare. Spanking children also might be thought to fall under this category, but spanking is for the *benefit* of the recipient in a way that capital punishment and just warfare are not.
9. Ibid., 140.

d. *Praise.* Scripture also commends conduct by praising it. We might think that it praises only those acts commanded by God, but I believe this category is larger than the last and overlaps some, but not all, of *b.* Consider David's mighty men, who risked their lives to bring him a drink of water from the well at Bethlehem (2 Sam. 23:13-17). The passage commends their bravery, yet I doubt if David's other soldiers were condemned for not risking their lives to bring David water. This behavior was commendable, but it was not universally commanded. Similarly, consider Paul's advice in 1 Corinthians 7:27f. about marriage. In effect, Paul commends those in the Corinthian situation who have renounced marriage, but he says explicitly that those who marry have not sinned. Thus, although the renunciation of marriage is praiseworthy, it is not commanded for all. Also consider the praise bestowed on the widow who gave the two mites (Luke 21:2): most likely she was giving more than a tithe, more than her legal duty. And see the references under *c, (H)* to self-sacrifice.

Our discussion of praise places us on somewhat controversial ground. Roman Catholic theology teaches that man can perform "works of supererogation," works that somehow go beyond the requirements of God's law and whose merit may be applied to the credit of others. Protestants, however, have denied this notion for the following reasons. (A) None of our good works are good enough to gain favor with God, and so certainly none of them are good enough to *exceed* God's standards. God's standard, ultimately, is the perfect righteousness of Christ, who was a perfect self-sacrifice. Not even David's mighty men measured up to that standard. (B) All of our good works are the result of God's grace working within us. (C) Whatever else we may say about praiseworthy actions, they do not earn merit for salvation, either for the one doing them or for anyone else. For these reasons, we must clearly distinguish "praiseworthy actions" from "works of supererogation."

More analysis is needed on the subject of praiseworthy actions. After all the qualifications have been made, however, we must recognize that there are actions that God praises whose omission is not always sinful. Are these actions obligatory? They are not obligatory for all; those who omit them may be acting righteously. But these actions may be obligatory for a particular individual. Certainly, in a way, David's mighty men felt *constrained* to do what they did. And Paul was "constrained" by the love of Christ to a life of great suffering (1 Cor. 9:16f.; 2 Cor. 5:14). Many who have expressed their love in self-sacrifice have testified to a profound sense of obligation that they could neither ignore nor refuse.

Where does such a sense of obligation come from? It comes from the biblical rule of *love*. Paul commands the Corinthian church to "eagerly desire the greater gifts" and then describes to them the "most excellent way" of self-sacrificing love (1 Cor. 12:31-13:13). We have an obligation increasingly to seek to love others as Jesus loves us (John 13:34f.; 15:12; 1 John 2:7-11; 3:11; 4:10-12). Different believers will show the love of Christ in different ways. David's mighty men risked their lives to get water from Bethlehem's well. The other soldiers, however, did not necessarily sin by failing to accompany them. Each of us will be called on in *some* way to deny himself, to take up his cross, and to follow Jesus.

How do we hear that call for self-denying discipleship? We hear it by learning from Scripture the *kinds* of actions God praises, by looking carefully at our opportunities and abilities (David's mighty men, doubtless, thought they would succeed), and by challenging our own complacency.[10]

Paul gave up certain "rights" (1 Cor. 9:4-15), and he did so by compulsion (v. 16). But there is no divine law that we give up our rights. If there were such a law, those "rights" wouldn't be rights at all! Paul was not compelled by any such law but by the love of Christ. And that love, that *compelling* love, moved him specifically to share the gospel with others (9:19, 20, 22). Paul knew that a certain kind of self-sacrifice would enable him to be more effective as an evangelist.[11] And having made that judgment, with God's help Paul overcame his own human (though not necessarily sinful) desires for comfort, marriage, and pleasure. He looked forward to the praise of Christ and to the "crown of righteousness" (2 Tim. 4:8).

---

10. Note the three perspectives!

11. Paul's sense of *purposiveness* in making such a self-sacrifice is important. God does not call us to self-sacrifice for its own sake; that would be meaningless asceticism.

C. SITUATIONAL COMPLICATIONS

The line between the preceding section and this one is not sharp. We have already discussed some of the various relations between norm and situation, and we have seen that using Scripture always involves a knowledge of the situation to which we wish to apply it. Therefore *any* ethical use of Scripture will be complicated to some extent by "situational factors."

Although the heading for this section is "Situational Complications," we are still discussing "principles" and "norms"; we are still discussing the "normative perspective." And although we will not discuss the "situational perspective" per se until chapter 3, since the three perspectives are actually inseparable, we must now discuss how situations affect, indeed complicate, our determination of ethical norms. For after all, we are seeking an *applied* norm, a norm that is situation-specific.

As we noted earlier, the concept of a "conflict of duties" is unscriptural. But because of the sheer difficulty of the ethical issues that we face in life, it is a plausible notion. The world *is* fallen, after all, as the advocates of conflict ethics emphasize, and often it presents us with no fully congenial alternatives. Two people are drowning, for example, and I must choose which one to save and which one to neglect—not a happy prospect. Although we never have to choose between two ethically *wrong actions* (as conflict ethics would have it), sometimes we have to choose between acting to remedy one *evil situation* or another; we have to choose between two *evils*, not between two *wrongs*. The two drowning swimmers are each in an evil situation, and our choice to rescue one of them may mean death to the other. Either choice, then, leaves someone in a condition of unalleviated harm, that is, evil. But in a situation where we cannot save both swimmers, either choice is righteous before God. Thus although there are two evil situations, we are not faced with a conflict of *duty* in choosing to save one swimmer and not the other.

Therefore even the Christian who rejects conflict ethics should recognize the need for careful thought when weighing decisions among evils. And in medical ethics, deciding among evil situations is commonplace. Medical ethics deals with cases of illness or injury whose treatment is almost always unpleasant or potentially dangerous in some way. Thus the unpleasantness or potential danger of one treatment must be weighed against another and against the unpleasant or potentially dangerous option of leaving the condition untreated.

Therefore we need to discuss the topic of "risk/benefit" or "cost/benefit" analysis. In the literature of medical ethics, the question of whether to use a certain treatment or to engage in certain research is answered by saying, "Yes, if the benefits outweigh the risks and/or costs." That answer, of course, is not an answer but only a further set of questions, and those questions can become extremely complex as distinctions multiply.

Books such as Beauchamp and Childress's *Principles of Biomedical Ethics* [12] and Childress's *Priorities in Biomedical Ethics* (Philadelphia: Westminster Press, 1981) [13] raise many valid issues that make it difficult, the authors realize, to quantify risk/benefit and cost/benefit ratios. There are many kinds of benefits to be weighed, and there are many kinds of risks and costs to be evaluated. The effectiveness of treatment is never certain; at best it is always a matter of probability that is subject to the possibility of harmful complications. To what extent should we accept a reduced benefit to decrease the risk? What criteria should we use to determine if a certain risk is acceptable? What role should economic considerations play? In terms of social expenditures, where is it best to invest our research funds? [14] Should such funds be invested in cancer research when any possible cure for this deadly disease seems so far away? Or should they be invested in research on arthritis, which is a less deadly but nevertheless quite painful disease that causes much suffering and against which more rapid progress seems likely? How can we quantify the value of preventing suffering when contrasted with the value of preventing death? What value should we assign to human life itself, especially in situations where the "quality" of that life is questionable? If by genetic engineering we could increase the intelligence of our offspring by 100 percent, would it be wise to do so?

12. Especially 135ff., 209ff.
13. Especially 105ff.
14. We will leave aside the question of the role of government versus that of private enterprise in such funding.

One can get dizzy mulling over risk/benefit and cost/benefit ratios of various medical treatments. Here the methodological haze is especially thick. The question is not only What are the answers? but How do we begin to look for answers? How would we find an answer, if one existed?

Our concern is to formulate an *evangelical* methodology in response to those questions: What difference does it make to trust in a fully authoritative Scripture? It is tempting to say that since Scripture does not address these matters specifically, they are *adiaphora* or "matters of Christian liberty": we can do what we like. The function of Scripture then would be to set us free from any pains of conscience in these areas. But in the light of our previous analysis of *adiaphora*, that alternative is not possible. Even in these difficult areas, God expects us to bring the broader principles of Scripture to bear. He wants us to do the *wisest* thing we can do, and wisdom is the art of applying God's truth to life's situations.

This does not mean that each of these problems in life has only one ethically correct answer. In medical ethics, as in other areas of life, some problems will leave us with a choice between several right, godly alternatives. Perhaps two or more answers will be ethically equal and good, though perhaps only one of them will be exceptionally praiseworthy.

What are some of the "broader biblical principles" that can help us analyze the risk/benefit and cost/benefit ratios of various medical treatments? Identifying these principles will help us see the methodological advantages of an evangelical position. Unfortunately, little work has been done by evangelicals in this area. Rather than seeking to develop distinctively biblical perspectives, much of their writing simply repeats what liberals and secularists have said. Although my thinking in this area is rudimentary, I suggest the following ways in which a distinctively biblical perspective may help us deal with the kinds of issues we have been discussing.

1. Scripture teaches us that God's world is meaningful and valuable. Therefore discussing what is meaningful and what is valuable is worthwhile. Since many people believe the world is meaningless and are suspicious of rational arguments, and since many others try to be rational without having a basis for being so, it is a considerable advantage to know that "meaning" and "value" exist.

2. Scripture also teaches that we should generally expect nature to be uniform, that we should expect regular conjunctions of cause and effect. That regularity allows us to make rough assessments of the consequences of our actions. Our assessments of such consequences, however, are not the ultimate grounds of our decisions, as in utilitarianism, though they are an important means for applying the principles of Scripture to situations.

3. Scripture gives us a proper perspective on the value of human life, which is the fundamental value on which all risk/benefit and cost/benefit analysis rests.

a. Because man is made in the image of God, human life is precious to God. No human being may take the life of another, except as authorized by Scripture (i.e., just capital punishment, war, self-defense).

b. At the same time, the sheer prolongation of physical life is not an absolute priority (John 10:11; 15:13; 2 Cor. 4-5 [esp. 5:6ff.]; 11:21-27; Phil. 1:20-26; 1 John 3:16). Other things are sometimes more important. It can be right, even praiseworthy (remember David's mighty men), to put one's life at risk for others. Physical death is not the end of life, and medical treatment is not our ultimate hope.

4. Earlier we discussed the "doctrine of carefulness": since even accidental killing is a crime in biblical law, and since Scripture forbids all actions or even attitudes (anger) that jeopardize human life, we must take great pains to avoid placing human life at risk. (See chapter 1, B, 9, a, above.) It is not always wrong to place one's *own* life at risk (above, 3), but it is always wrong to put *someone else's* life at risk. We must, therefore, distinguish between treatment that is voluntary (in which the patient gives his informed consent: see chapter 2, C) and involuntary treatment (such as in a medical emergency, when a patient is unconscious and there is no competent proxy).

Now of course nearly every medical treatment involves some risk to the patient's life, but illness and injury involve risk as well, risk that is greater in the absence of treatment. So we cannot adopt the principle that there is to be no risk at all. We must be concerned, however, about medical treatments that *increase* risk beyond the risk involved in leaving the problem untreated.

A patient may voluntarily undergo such an increased level of risk. Imagine a church organist whose hand coordination has been destroyed by disease of the nervous system. His life, however, is not threatened, and he can otherwise live a normal life. I can imagine the love of Christ constraining him to accept a risky medical treatment to restore coordination, with the goal of again using his most important gift for God. That could, in some circumstances (if the man had no dependents, for example), be a praiseworthy decision.

Even in more "ordinary" situations, we often accept increased levels of risk. Those who work in coal mines and in law enforcement, for example, voluntarily increase their level of risk. And it would certainly not be wrong to accept corresponding levels of risk in medical treatment. But there are limits. To increase one's risk without adequate and compensating corresponding benefits would be suicidal. I often wonder if much cosmetic surgery should be rejected under this criterion. Should a woman subject herself to the stress of surgery merely to increase the size of her breasts?

When treatment is *involuntary*, however, I would contend that a physician should not put a patient at risk beyond the risk involved in leaving the problem untreated. This principle would rule out most abortions, (1) since the operation often increases the danger to the woman beyond the risk of childbirth and (2) since it always (infinitely, one might say) increases the danger to the child, except in cases like ectopic pregnancy when it is clear that the child will die anyway.

5. "Quality of life" judgments, however inappropriate they may be in terminal cases (see chapter 2, B, C, Appendix A), certainly play a legitimate role in many medical decisions. Scripture tells us much about the quality of life that is best for human beings. The best life is a life lived in fellowship with God.

a. Therefore treating an unbelieving terminal patient should leave the broadest possible opportunity for evangelism. Isolation and mind-numbing drugs should be minimized.[15]

b. Believing patients should have the fullest possible access to the means of grace—the Scriptures, fellowship with other Chris-

---

15. Payne's emphasis on this point is excellent; see his index for references to *evangelism*.

tians, and the support of family and church. The spiritual dimensions of healing ought to be fully pursued.[16] James 5:14-16 assures us that the church plays an indispensable role in healing. Whether one takes the "anointing" as the administration of first-century medicine or as an "unction" ceremony in which divine intervention is sought, it is clear that the elders of the church have a significant responsibility for the treatment of the patient.

c. Godliness is more important than physical healing. A physician should never assist a patient in an immoral act, whether by performing an abortion or by helping a teen-age girl hide her promiscuous sex life from her parents.

d. The physically handicapped who know and love God enjoy a higher quality of life, in the final analysis, than "normal" people who do not, but a physical handicap per se is never a ground for nontreatment.

6. Scripture gives us guidelines about the nature of disease and healing. Because diseases entered the world as a result of the Fall, diseases are a result of sin, though a given individual's diseases are not *necessarily* a punishment for his or her sins. But because an individual's diseases *can be* a result of or a punishment for his or her sins, regeneration and sanctification can be instrumental in healing and in preventing illness.[17] Not only is godliness more important than physical healing (above, 5), it is also an important *means* of healing. Furthermore, the ministries of prayer, Christian counselling, and fellowship are as important to healing as is medical treatment and should be taken into account as "benefits" whenever "risk/benefit" relationships are discussed.

7. The economic costs of healing—questions of cost/benefit—also should be examined from a biblical perspective. Generally speaking, human life is more important than economic wealth. Scripture is eloquent about the folly of trusting in riches and of using wealth without compassion for others. Therefore when a man's family, for example, refuses to pay for medical treatment that could save his life, they must, to say the least, sustain a heavy burden of proof. This is especially true in view of the family's central role in providing for human welfare: "If anyone does not provide for his

16. This is another strength of Payne's discussion; see especially chapters 5-8.
17. Ibid., 75ff.

relatives, and especially for his immediate family, he has denied the faith and is worse than an unbeliever" (1 Tim. 5:8). At the same time, we should recognize the possibility that either (a) the family simply doesn't *have* the money for an expensive operation and may have no means of getting it, or (b) to pay for such an operation would mean that other family responsibilities (needs, not wants) could not be met.

Thus when considering the economic costs of healing, there is some room for deliberation, for weighing alternatives. In some cases, for a patient to refuse treatment for economic reasons could be a godly form of self-sacrifice. For example, precisely because of 1 Timothy 5:8, a man might refuse a treatment because it would bankrupt his family (and possibly the church diaconate as well). But what if such a person is incompetent to make that decision? May the family, or other proxies, make the decision for him? I do not believe that anyone has the right to force someone to make a sacrifice without that person's consent (see below). If economics were the only issue, then the recommended treatment should be provided. Who should pay for such treatment if the family cannot and there is no insurance? According to Scripture, in such cases that financial responsibility rests on others in society. In the Old Testament, neglect of the poor is a national sin; and according to Old Testament law, everyone (presumably everyone who can) was expected to be willing to make loans to the poor (Exod. 22:25ff.; Deut. 15:7-11; Pss. 37:26; 112:5; Prov. 19:17). And the New Testament mandates an equal willingness to share financial resources (Acts 2:45ff.; 2 Cor. 8-9; Gal. 2:10; Eph. 4:28; James 2:2ff.). That is not to say that such benevolence should be administered by the state; those texts don't say that. But society does have a responsibility to bear the medical costs of the poor and needy, and certainly Christians should provide this sort of care for one another.[18]

18. I realize there are many unanswered questions here. Readers have asked "How will society be organized to meet these needs, if the state is not to do it?" "Who will decide who receives and who does not receive treatment when that treatment cannot be given to all who need it?" Ideally, all society would be Christian and there would be one Christian church whose deacons would administer all such funds and whose elders would make the necessary decisions. In the absence of such unity, however, piecemeal methods must be used: charitable societies, cooperation among churches and denominations, Christians in a neighborhood or a city sharing their funds. But others are better equipped to answer the "how" question than I am.

8. On questions of social priorities for medical research (e.g., arthritis research versus cancer research), I think Scripture gives us considerable individual freedom. In Scripture the responsibility for health and welfare is not given to a central agency (certainly not to government), and so there is no single organization that is competent to define social priorities in this area. Social priorities for medical research should be the sum total of the priorities of individuals and of smaller groups (e.g., church sessions).

How then should individuals decide where to place their resources? The question is a subtle one. Scripture does not require us to invest our resources *only* in that which is objectively most important. God Himself, the supremely important one, demands only a tithe of our wealth (though He demands all of our devotion). And one need not believe that agriculture is more important than plumbing to become a farmer rather than a plumber. To an extent, within the constraints of God's law, we may invest our resources freely on what strikes our fancy.

Nevertheless, there are some objective limits. It would be perverse to spend church benevolence money on hangnail research. Our decisions must be guided by godly *wisdom*, the application of God's Word to situations. And generally speaking, the question of investment in research is not a question about general divine commands or prohibitions but about what investments in a particular situation are "praiseworthy." What investments, in other words, best display the love of Christ? (Recall our discussion in chapter 1, B, 9, d, above, as to how such decisions are made.) Although individual Christians with their different experiences, burdens, concerns, and interests will answer the question differently, I believe that there will be a discernible unity amid the differences, a unity that emerges from the sincere intention of all Christians to make the *wisest* use of God's money.

D. EXISTENTIAL INSIGHT

Although we are still talking about the normative perspective, we have not been able to avoid reference to the other two perspectives. The situational perspective must be taken into account whenever we formulate our norms, because the norms of medical ethics are always *applied* norms; they are norms that relate to, that are applied to, real-life situations and questions. They are not norms about theoretical problems and hypothetical cases. Similarly, when discussing norms we cannot avoid reference to the existential perspective, because the existential perspective describes the process by which *we* come to appropriate such norms for ourselves; it describes how *we* come to know them, to delight in them, and to obey them. Understanding the *personal process* by which we appropriate norms is a necessary condition for being able to learn what those norms are, because ethical norms apply to and are appropriated by persons. Note also that each norm requires its own joyful acceptance; obeying a norm out of a mere grudging acceptance is something less than the full biblical requirement. Thus there is a close relation between "norm" and "appropriation."

Because we need to discuss the existential perspective as it bears on the normative perspective, we must discuss *conscience*, one of the means by which we gain ethical knowledge, and *motive*, the interior and deepest dimension of the human act itself.

1. According to Scripture, *conscience* is a function of the *heart* (cf. 2 Sam. 24:10), and the "heart" is the religious center of a human being from which flows all the issues of life. Thus the "heart" is not a "part" of us; it is our whole self viewed from a particular perspective. To say "my conscience knows" something is simply to say that "I" know it, in the depths of my being, in my heart. Thus ethical knowledge is a function of the whole person (Acts 23:1; 24:16; Rom. 9:1; 13:5; 1 Cor. 8:7-12; 10:25-29 in context; 1 Tim. 1:5), and conscience is that "faculty," that capacity or ability, by means of which we come to discern good and evil (Heb. 5:14).

Conscience is not infallible, for we are not infallible. Scripture describes conscience as infected by sin (1 Cor. 8:7, 12; 1 Tim. 4:2; Titus 1:15). It can be "seared" by continued disregard for and violation of God's will, but it can never, I believe, be completely eradicated. According to Romans 1, even the worst unbelievers know God's standards; and because of that, God continues to address their consciences.

To "follow your conscience," then, is nothing less than to seek to follow God's law. Conscience is not a norm to itself, over and above the law; it is a human means of learning and obeying the law itself. It is always wrong to disobey conscience—not because conscience is divine but because to "disobey conscience" is to disobey what we think God is saying to us. So disobedience to conscience always involves a rebellious heart.

Conscience operates by applying God's Word to situations. Therefore conscience is trained not only by studying God's Word but also by our experience of discipleship (Heb. 5:12-15), by our experience in applying God's Word to our lives, and by our experience of Christian warfare. Ethical knowledge, then, is not merely an academic achievement; it is a result of regeneration and sanctification; it is a product of the Christian life.[19]

Therefore growth in ethical knowledge can be a mysterious process, like learning to recognize patterns in an optical illusion (e.g., the "duck-rabbit" or the inverted staircase). Gradually we learn to call things in our experience by their biblical names. For example, we learn that sex outside of marriage is adultery, not "recreational sex," that abortion is murder, not the "extraction of products of conception." We are like King David, who had to learn to recognize adultery and murder for what they were, after his heart (his conscience) had grown cold. For David, the "light dawned" through a prophetic parable. For us, the "light" of ethical knowledge may "dawn" through any number of mysterious ways. Ethical knowledge is not always the product of rational argument, but it does always reflect the working of the Spirit, whose ways are often mysterious (John 3:8). We can hear rational arguments, but what makes us *accept* them?

In the midst of all the complicated arguments of medical ethics, it is too easy to think that we can never reach an assured conclusion. And when that is the case, it is important to remember that persuasion and assurance are essentially the results of supernatural acts of God. And we should also remember that Scripture contains a clear (though not always rationally comprehensible) methodology for attaining this certainty. Paul states that methodology this

---

19. Cf. what Jesus says about *doctrinal* knowledge in John 7:17. Many have said that "life is built upon doctrine"; but there is also a sense in which the reverse is true.

way: "Be not conformed to this world, but be transformed by the renewal of your mind, that you will be able to prove the good, pleasing and perfect will of God" (Rom. 12:2).[20]

2. A *motive* is the inward ground of someone's decision or action. It can be an attitude, like fear or love, or it can be a goal that is capable of articulation ("I'm doing it to earn money"). Motives are the grounds of our acts, as well as part of our actions. Actions begin with motives, and motives are the most rudimentary part, the essence, of acts. Why? Once an attitude or a goal becomes a motive, the decision to act has been made, whether or not the act is successfully executed.[21] Therefore, in view of Matthew 5:27ff., a motive or intention to commit a sin, even if that intention never comes to fruition, is just as blameworthy as the sin itself. Therefore from a biblical perspective, we may say that motives are the interior and deepest dimension of acts.

Scripture demands pure motives, for it demands nothing less than a righteous heart, that is, righteousness at the deepest level of our being (Deut. 6:5; Jer. 31:33ff.; Matt. 5:8; etc.). Scripture condemns externalism and hypocrisy (Isa. 29:13f.; Matt. 23) and requires faith (Rom. 14:23) and love (1 Cor. 13:1-3) as necessary conditions for any good work. Faith and love also are sufficient conditions for any good work: love fulfills the law (John 14:15, 21; 15:10; Rom. 13:10; 1 John 2:3-5; etc.), and true faith does good works (Gal. 5:6; James 2:14-26). Thus it is inconceivable that any act motivated by true love or by true faith could be evil.

Sometimes it is said that good motives do not render actions acceptable,[22] and that is true at one level. One certainly cannot *excuse* a sin by saying it was done out of love (this is a common claim in cases of adultery and euthanasia), because in such cases both the act and the motive are defective, whatever the perpetrator may *claim*

20. For a more secular, concise approach to the concept of conscience, see Beauchamp and Childress, 237ff.

21. For example, once my goal to make money becomes a motive to rob a bank, the robbery has already been decided on, whether or not the robbery itself is ever carried out. Even if the robbery never takes place, another ethically wrong act already has, that is, the act of *deciding* to rob. And that is what we mean by "motive." You can't have a motive without an act that it motivates, whether or not that act is observable. You cannot have a motive unless it is a motive *of something*.

22. E.g., Beauchamp and Childress, 234.

about his or her motives. Furthermore, the argument from good motive to good act works only in connection with the most *basic* human motives. Where lesser motives are in view (e.g., "I robbed him because I needed to buy food for my family"), a good motive does not necessarily imply a good act. But when one's most fundamental motive is truly blameless (a motive for Christian love), the act also will be blameless. He who has a legitimate motive always does God's will. There is, therefore, a sense in which a good motive *does* render actions acceptable. "Good motive," as we saw earlier, is the essence of every good act. Like "obedient to the law" and "appropriate to the situation," "good motive" is a "perspective" on every good work.

Because an examination of motives provides an additional criterion (or an additional form of the one criterion) to use in evaluating actions, we will now discuss the existential perspective under the normative! The existential perspective serves as a valuable check and balance to our thinking. I have known some people who seemed immune to the traditional arguments against abortion who came to an anti-abortion position when they realized the enormous *selfishness* of the act.

One prominent topic in the literature of medical ethics where discussions of motive (i.e., "intent") play a major role is the "principle of double effect." The "principle of double effect" states that a procedure leading to a harmful effect can be justified if "the harmful effect is seen as an indirect or merely foreseen effect, not the direct and intended effect of the action."[23] For example, Roman Catholic theology condemns abortion, but in two situations it justifies physicians' actions that kill fetuses: removal of a cancerous uterus and terminating an ectopic pregnancy. According to this argument, when a physician removes a cancerous uterus, he does not *intend* to destroy the fetus, though that is always the result, indeed the foreseen result. Beauchamp and Childress note the following four conditions that must be the case for the "principle of double effect" to be a justifiable one.

23. Ibid., 102.

(A) The action in itself must be good or at least morally indifferent.

(B) The agent must intend only the good effect and not the evil effect. The evil effect is foreseen, not intended. . . .

(C) The evil effect cannot be a *means* to the good effect. . . .[24]

(D) There must be a proportionality between the good and evil effects of the action.[25]

But there are problems with the "principle of double effect." Principle (C), for example, has been thought to rule out a fetal craniotomy (crushing the baby's head) to save a woman in labor. Many, however, have asked whether there is any significant moral difference between a fetal craniotomy and removing the uterus of a pregnant woman. The *intentions* in both cases seem similar; in a craniotomy the death of the fetus may not be wanted or desired (except as an unfortunate means), and it may be genuinely regretted. In my opinion, the attempt to justify removing a uterus by appealing to intention is not cogent. Acts can be justified by intention only at the level of *ultimate* intention, and that is not the case in the argument before us. Therefore I think that the two actions, craniotomy and uterus removal, are on the same moral level: either both can be justified or neither can be justified. I am prepared to justify either action *if* it can be shown that either is truly necessary to save the mother's life, and my ground for doing so is that Scripture warrants self-defense (Exod. 22:2; Deut. 20; Rom. 13).

For similar reasons, arguments about intentions are rarely, if ever, decisive in ethical disputes, especially in a practical field like medicine, where we tend to think more about immediate intentions than about ultimate ones. Still, intention is an important perspective when we search our *own* consciences. Observing the presence within ourselves of ungodly motives can, if we are spiritually sensitive, interrupt us from following ungodly courses of action.

24. The point here is that the end does not justify the means; we should not do evil that good may come.
25. Beauchamp and Childress, 103.

In the foregoing manner, then, all three perspectives assist us to discern ethical norms. And of course the quest for ethical norms is inseparable from the work of putting those norms into practice. Therefore our discussion must now become more practical, focusing first upon the patient and then upon various specific situations.

2

THE EXISTENTIAL PERSPECTIVE: FOCUS ON THE PATIENT

The existential perspective, which we touched on in the last section, focuses on the moral agent, the decision maker. In medical treatment the decision maker is generally the patient, who usually is advised by physicians, family, friends, counsellors, the church, and so on. There are, however, important cases in which the patient is incompetent, and decisions about his welfare must be made by others. In such cases the actual decision makers are supposed to act in the best interests of the patient, to serve as proxies for him or for her. Thus in considering the existential perspective, we will focus on the patient's rights and dignity.

A. PERSONHOOD

Christianity is profoundly personalistic. Unlike secularists, who believe that the personal aspects of the universe are the result of impersonal forces, Christians believe that the impersonal aspects of the universe were created by the personal God of Scripture. And Christians believe that God created man as His image, that we are profoundly like God. Therefore the highest principle of Christian ethics, love for God and for one another, is also distinctively personal. Thus a Christian understanding of medical ethics will emphasize the importance of treating "patients as persons."[1]

And that raises the questions: What is a person? How do we define personhood and personality? There has been no shortage of attempts to define *personality* for ethical purposes.[2] Lewis P. Bird, for example, in quoting characterizations from Robert L. Sinsheimer, says that humanity is "our self-awareness, our perception of past, present and future, . . . our drive to reduce the role of Fate in human affairs. . . ."[3] He also notes some criteria from Joseph Fletcher.[4] On the criterion of "minimal intelligence," Fletcher says, "Any individual . . . who falls below the I.Q. 40-mark in a standard Stanford-Binet test, amplified if you like by other tests, is unquestionably a person; below the 20-mark, not a person." And Fletcher suggests the following additional criteria for defining personhood: "control of existence," "curiosity," "balance of rationality and feeling," and "euphoria and affectionate responses to caresses." Even Lewis Smedes of the Christian Reformed Church and Fuller Seminary speaks of "bodies without persons," though his criteria of personhood are evidently not as narrow as Fletcher's.[5]

It's not wrong to try to discern those distinctive qualities that separate human beings from the animal kingdom. It is wrong, however, to use such speculations as the basis for denying some

1. Echoing the title of an important book by Paul Ramsey, *The Patient as Person* (New Haven: Yale University Press, 1970).

2. From a Christian perspective, the relation between "image of God" and "person" is that being the image of God is the ground for having the rights of a person.

3. Lewis P. Bird, "Dilemmas in Biomedical Ethics," in Carl F. H. Henry, ed., *Horizons of Science* (San Francisco: Harper and Row, 1978), 135. He quotes Robert L. Sinsheimer, "Prospects for Future Scientific Developments: Ambush or Opportunity?" in Bruce Hilton et al., eds., *Ethical Issues in Human Genetics* (New York: Plenum Press, 1973).

4. Bird, 135, quoting Fletcher, "Indicators of Humanhood," 2 *The Hastings Center Report* (November 1972): 1-4.

5. Lewis Smedes, *Mere Morality* (Grand Rapids: Wm. B. Eerdmans Publishing Co., 1983), 148f.

human beings the rights of persons, to oppress those whom we do not recognize as "fully human." That was the great crime of the Nazis, and it is a crime that is perpetrated daily against unborn children and regularly against handicapped infants.

Scripture never defines the image of God in terms of specific qualities or abilities. Instead, Scripture teaches that *human beings as such* are individually created in God's image (Gen. 1:26, 27; 9:6; 1 Cor. 11:7; James 3:9)[6] and that a "human being" is anyone who belongs to the race of Adam (Gen. 5:1-3ff.).[7] Thus everyone who belongs to the race of Adam bears God's image (cf. Gen. 5:1-3ff.). Because being the image of God is the scriptural ground for having the rights of a person (Gen. 9:6; James 3:9), we can say that Scripture equates "being God's image" with "being a person." That scriptural understanding of "image of God" and of "person" can raise difficult questions. Precisely how, we may ask, is an anencephalic child God's image? In what sense is that child a person? Although we may not be able to answer such questions,[8] in Genesis 9:6 and in James 3:9, Scripture commands us to respect the image of God. And the contexts of those verses absolutely exclude any attempt to distinguish persons from nonpersons within the human race. James 3:9, for example, addresses a situation in which some people understood the image of God too narrowly. According to James, the solution to that too narrow perspective was not to recognize "criteria of personhood" but to regard *all* humans ("men" in the text) as God's image.

B. THE PRINCIPLE OF "AUTONOMY"

In the literature of medical ethics, a patient's dignity as a person is often said to mandate respect for his or her "autonomy." According to Beauchamp and Childress, for example,

6. See, for example, G. C. Berkouwer, *Man: The Image of God* (Grand Rapids: Wm. B. Eerdmans Publishing Co., 1962).

7. In Genesis 1:26-27 and 5:1, Scripture uses *man* to mean "human being."

8. Meredith G. Kline, *Images of the Spirit* (Grand Rapids: Baker Book House, 1980), and John Murray, *Collected Writings* 4 vols. (Edinburgh: The Banner of Truth Trust, 1977), 2:34ff., however, recognize physical, as well as mental, aspects to the "image."

Autonomy is a form of personal liberty of action where the individual determines his or her own course of action in accordance with a plan chosen by himself or herself.[9]

To respect a person's autonomy, they assert, is to recognize that

Insofar as an autonomous agent's actions do not infringe the autonomous actions of others, that person should be free to perform whatever action he wishes—even if it involves serious risk for the agent and even if others consider it to be foolish.[10]

Beauchamp and Childress recognize that the principle of autonomy is not absolute or applicable to all situations.

Some persons are not in a position to act in a sufficiently autonomous manner, perhaps because they are immature, incapacitated, ignorant, coerced, or in a position in which they can be exploited by others. Infants and irrationally suicidal individuals are typical examples.[11]

The authors also recognize the legitimacy of interfering with competent agents when the autonomous choices of those agents would be harmful to third parties or would violate other moral principles,[12] and on that basis they justify what they call "weak paternalism." "Weak paternalism" also is used to justify temporary intervention in cases where the competence of the patient is uncertain.[13] As a rule, however, Beauchamp and Childress insist that it is wrong to violate the autonomy of a competent patient, "merely for his/her own good," which would be "strong paternalism."[14]

9. Tom L. Beauchamp and James F. Childress, *Principles of Biomedical Ethics* (New York: Oxford University Press, 1979), 56.
10. Ibid., 59.
11. Ibid., 60.
12. Ibid., 159ff.; James F. Childress, *Priorities in Biomedical Ethics* (Philadelphia: Westminster Press, 1981), 23ff.
13. Beauchamp and Childress, 161.
14. They do, however, suggest that there are individual cases where even a strong paternalism is not inherently immoral (see 164 and Childress, 60). But the possibility of abuse leads them to reject strong paternalism as a *rule*, and that seems inconsistent with the general thrust of their argument (see below).

Beauchamp and Childress typically analyze cases where strong paternalism appears to be justified as cases of weak paternalism. One of their examples concerns a psychiatrist and his patient, a religious fanatic. The psychiatrist does not tell the patient the truth about his condition for fear the patient will maim himself. In effect, Beauchamp and Childress argue, the psychiatrist questioned the patient's competence, which made the psychiatrist's intervention weak, not strong, paternalism.[15] Childress mentions John Stuart Mill's argument that one should intervene to prevent a man from selling himself into slavery, even though his act is voluntary.[16] Childress accepts that position by arguing that assessments of risk/benefit may sometimes take precedence over informed consent. On the basis of that principle, Childress argues that it would not be right to prevent a man from climbing a dangerous mountain, though it would not necessarily be wrong to refuse him a dangerous medical procedure that he wished to risk. As with a man who desires to sell himself into slavery, Childress argues, by allowing a patient to determine a medical procedure, "the danger of exploitation is too great."[17] I judge this to be a case of *strong* paternalism, contrary to the general view of Beauchamp and Childress.

That last illustration suggests a weakness in the whole discussion of strong and weak paternalism. Couldn't most medical interventions, even those in the strong paternalism category, be justified with the argument Childress used to justify withholding a medical procedure? And even if one restricts interventions to cases of weak paternalism, couldn't *any* intervention be justified as weak, given a particular set of values? Soviet psychiatrists confine political dissidents to mental hospitals against their will on the ground that anyone who engages in dissent against the state must be incompetent to make his own decisions. At the other extreme, advocates of suicide generally argue that competent people do indeed sometimes engage in such acts and therefore should not be prevented from doing so.[18] The philosophical arguments offered for this view are drawn from Kant and Mill, not from Scripture.[19] That fact doesn't refute the

15. Beauchamp and Childress, 160f.
16. Childress, 60f.
17. Ibid.
18. See discussion in ibid., 85ff.
19. Ibid., 56ff.

principle, but it doesn't recommend it to Evangelicals. What does Scripture say about autonomy and the criteria of competence?

The word *autonomy* should be rejected, since it almost invariably connotes lawlessness, which is the opposite of man's responsibility to God.[20] But the idea that competent persons under God have the right to make their own decisions about medical treatment is certainly scriptural. Although all of us are subject to human authorities (parents, church, state, schools, employers, and so forth), their dominion and areas of jurisdiction are limited. None of them has the right to make medical decisions for competent patients.[21] But what about incompetent patients such as children? The authority of parents over children is comprehensive under God. Parents function as prophets, priests, and kings and as school, church, and state to their children. Parents are responsible for their children's welfare, and parental authority is comprehensive and unquestionable, unless used to command a violation of God's law. Like children, other incompetents in Scripture were placed in quasi-family environments.[22] In the Old and New Testaments, persons who for physical or mental reasons had lost their competence to make decisions were cared for within a family context and were subject to the authority structure of the family. Nevertheless, no family is absolutely free to impose its will on one of diminished capacity. In the Bible, even slave owners were limited in the discipline they could impose on their slaves (Exod. 21:20, 26f.; Eph. 6:9). Furthermore, sometimes a family itself exercises authority in an incompetent fashion.

In Scripture, the church also plays an important role in assisting those whose judgment is not fully competent. The line between family and church is not a sharp one, because the church is like an

20. I would rather speak of "personal responsibility."

21. And certainly Scripture does not anoint the medical profession as an independent authority alongside these others, though medical expertise, like all wisdom, is to be respected. See Proverbs 1:1-7, 20-33; 2:1-4:27, passim.

22. Perhaps this is how we are to understand the Old Testament legislation about slavery: One who lives irresponsibly is sentenced to a "second childhood" under quasi-parental authority to learn habits of godly responsibility. See James B. Jordan, *The Law of the Covenant: An Exposition of Exodus 21-23* (Tyler, Tex.: Institute for Christian Economics, 1984), 88-89.

extended family, the family of God. Israel, the Old Testament people of God, was essentially a family, the descendants of Abraham, Isaac, and Jacob, though this family was open to those outside the physical family who wished to confess the true God. In the New Testament, believers are "brothers and sisters" (Acts 1:16; 6:3; 11:1; 12:17; Rom. 1:13 and regularly throughout). They are the "mother and brothers" of Jesus (Matt. 12:49), they are the new family that God gives to us when we forsake all else for Jesus (Mark 10:30). Note also the analogy between family and church that is implicit in the qualifications for church office (1 Tim. 3:5; Titus 1:6). Family and church have similar functions: fellowship, teaching, discipline, welfare, worship, witness.

In the church, as in the family, believers bear one another's burdens. When one suffers, the others suffer with him (1 Cor. 12:26). The church, especially its elders, plays an important role in healing (James 5:14-18). The church also plays a role in making *judgments* in cases of disputes; in 1 Corinthians 6:1-8 Paul teaches that for Christians the church should take the place of civil courts. Believers are not to go to court before unbelievers but before representatives of the church. When we add these data together, it is clearly appropriate that the church, represented by its elders, plays a role in determining the proper treatment of an incompetent patient. This becomes especially important where the nuclear family is either nonexistent or incompetent. And even where the family is competent, as much as possible they should act in consultation with the church. Indeed, from a Christian perspective, a family that will not hear the church is by definition incompetent (Matt. 18:17).

This role of the church is not often recognized by the legal and medical establishments. It should be.[23]

Scripture also addresses the all-important question of the criteria of competence. Unlike the criteria used to judge competence in the U.S.S.R., according to the Bible, an active belief in God or in political freedom is not a ground of incompetence! The Bible defines competence in moral, spiritual, physical, and mental terms:

23. Historically, the church has played a major role in founding and administering hospitals. The discussion above indicates some of the reasons that this role for the church is appropriate. Also see George Grant, *The Dispossessed* (Westchester, Ill.: Crossway Books, 1986), 67f., 169-82.

competence is conformity to God's will. For example, according to the Bible, those who wish to take their lives seek to violate God's standards and thus are not fully competent. Physicians should not help such persons carry out their suicidal intentions, and all who are involved with such persons should take every necessary step to prevent them from killing themselves.

Let's look at several cases to see how scriptural principles of competence apply.

(i) A physician determines that an unconscious patient requires a certain treatment, but there are no family members available to give their consent and the patient does not belong to a church. What should the physician do? In the light of the parable of the Good Samaritan (Luke 10:25-37), I believe that he should proceed with the treatment he thinks most appropriate. Why? Because God's providence has placed him, in effect, *in loco parentis*, in the position of a parent. Although legal concerns currently inhibit such spontaneous decisions, the law should sanction, not discourage, that kind of effort to save life.

(ii) Following an automobile accident, a Jehovah's Witness refuses a blood transfusion for himself and for his daughter.[24] Should the physician transfuse them anyway? On moral and spiritual grounds, the adult patient's false view of God's will places his competence in question. And that spiritual ignorance, I believe, disqualifies him from determining the best treatment for his daughter. Her life should not be jeopardized because of his false theology. The physician, supported by church and civil courts if necessary, should transfuse the daughter.

What about the adult? Let's look at two possible situations. First, let's assume that the adult is unconscious, in a hospital bed, and so under the *de facto* care of an attending physician.[25] If the attending physician believes a transfusion is necessary to save the patient's life, then I believe that the physician should transfuse the patient and that there should be no legal barriers to his doing so. Like case

24. For religious reasons, Jehovah's Witnesses do not believe in receiving blood transfusions.

25. In this case, knowledge of the patient's antitransfusion convictions could have come from a note in his wallet or from a third party.

(i), this situation is analogous to that of the parable of the Good Samaritan. No physician should be penalized for making a responsible (i.e., godly) judgment about the needs of a patient. Second, let's assume that the adult is conscious and refuses treatment. In this case, his wish should be respected, because neither the physician nor the state has a divine mandate to impose treatment on someone by force, and imposing treatment by force requires nothing less than a divine mandate.

(iii) A patient demands a treatment that the physician thinks is not in the patient's best interest. What should the physician do? The physician clearly has a right to refuse the treatment, because it is the *physician's* personal responsibility ("autonomy") that is at issue. He may never be forced to give treatment that contradicts his conscience (e.g., abortion) or what he believes is in the patient's best interest.

C. INFORMED CONSENT AND DISCLOSURE

Recent medical ethics literature places particular importance on the idea of "informed consent" as an aspect of genuine patient "autonomy." Talk about a patient making his own decisions is empty unless the patient is given adequate information on which to base those decisions. Personal responsibility is also impaired if the decision is made under undue pressure.

"Adequate information" is commonly said to include "contemplated procedures, alternative available procedures, anticipated risks and benefits, and a statement offering the person an opportunity to ask further questions and to withdraw at any time (in the case of research)," though other factors are also mentioned in individual situations. "Adequate information" would include both "what a reasonable person would want to know" about the procedure and also "what the particular patient actually wants to know."[26] Not only must physicians offer and provide such information, but patients must be able to understand it and willing to act on it, if the "informed consent" requirement is to be fully met.

26. Beauchamp and Childress, 70ff.

"Undue pressure" or "coercion" would include threats of harm (physical, psychological, economic, etc.), promises of excessive reward, and the use of irrational persuasion techniques.[27] But these pressures are matters of degree. Patients are always subject to *some* influence in their decision-making processes. The question is How much is too much? That is, What is excessive influence? When does "influence" become "coercion"? From a Christian viewpoint, this is an area where spiritual discernment is especially needed.

Informed consent is an aspect of "autonomy," of personal responsibility, and like that broader principle, it pertains only to competent subjects. In the case of incompetent patients, families should make medical decisions in consultation with the physician and the church elders, when those families and elders are competent and available. Otherwise, the patient is under the *de facto* guardianship of the physician, who must make decisions on the basis of his expertise and according to the patient's best interests. Informed consent applies to the final decision maker, whomever that may be.

Sometimes, however, it is questionable whether any proxy is qualified to make a decision without the informed consent of the patient. That is true in the Saikewicz case, with which we began the book. It is also true in the case of a thirty-five-year-old, institutionalized, mentally retarded man who is being considered as a donor for a kidney transplant.[28] Assume that the potential donor is the closest possible genetic match to the intended recipient and that the intended recipient will die unless he receives a kidney from the potential donor. Should those involved seek a court order to force the transplant? I do not believe so. Although I believe that sometimes it is right to try and *heal* people without their informed consent (see the next paragraph), I do not believe that it is ever right to require extraordinary sacrifices of them without their permission.[29] Because I would not want someone to do that to me, on the basis of the Golden Rule, I reject such treatment of anyone else. Sometimes, then, the principle of informed consent takes precedence over other principles of medical ethics.

27. Ibid., 81.
28. Ibid., 176f.
29. See my earlier discussion on this point in chapter 1.

There are, however, some limitations to the principle of informed consent. First, as I mentioned in the last section, the model of the Good Samaritan is important. It shows that requirements for informed consent should not hinder giving spontaneous, uninhibited care to those in need. Second, like autonomy, informed consent is a necessary but not a sufficient condition of treatment. A physician should refuse treatment that he believes is not in a patient's best interest, even if the patient has given informed consent.

The biblical warrant for requiring informed consent is Scripture's command to be truthful to one another (Exod. 20:16; Eph. 4:25) and the principle of personal responsibility that we discussed earlier. Scripture does not require us to tell the *whole* truth, unless giving the partial truth would deceive.[30] There are, I believe, some situations in medicine where intentional nondisclosure is legitimate. Information that is not relevant to the treatment in question or that may only complicate the explanation without increasing the patient's knowledge should be omitted. What if a patient asks *not* to know his condition? In my view, that request must be judged incompetent. It is in the patient's best interest to know his condition, whether he wants to or not, especially when the news is the worst. Patients do better when given the truth.[31] Furthermore, if his case is terminal, a responsible patient will want to know so that he can properly arrange his affairs. And an unbelieving patient needs to know the truth about his condition so that he may be aware of his need for God.

Failing to disclose a patient's problem for fear that he will become anxious or suicidal is not warranted for at least two reasons. First, a physician cannot predict how a patient will respond to bad news. Second, a physician should assume that a patient will respond well; the patient should be given the benefit of the doubt.[32]

The question of disclosure has arisen in an acute way in association with the XYY chromosome pattern in males, which has tenta-

30. See John Murray, *Principles of Conduct* (Grand Rapids: Wm. B. Eerdmans Publishing Co., 1957), 125ff.

31. See Franklin Payne, *Biblical/Medical Ethics* (Milford, Mich.: Mott Media, 1985), 118, and the study that he cites to this effect.

32. Scripture calls us to assume the best of one another. No accusation is to be heard unless it is validated by two or three witnesses (Deut. 17:6ff.; Matt. 18:16; 2 Cor. 13:1; 1 Tim. 5:19).

tively been related to a higher incidence of criminal behavior. If a physician discovers this pattern in a young boy (perhaps in the course of investigating something else), should he tell the parents? Arguments against disclosure make the point that revealing the information might result in treating the boy as a young criminal, which would be harmful to him. I believe the physician should disclose the information: If the parents are otherwise competent, they should be given the benefit of the doubt. They should be taught clearly that the XYY pattern does not *determine* criminal behavior, at most it *predisposes* a person to act in certain ways.[33] Understanding that such a predisposition is possible may make the parents even more conscientious in their training and discipline of the boy.[34]

Should a potential birth defect in the unborn fetus of a pregnant woman whose pro-abortion sympathies are known be revealed to her? Absolutely not. Scripture warrants nondisclosure, even deceit, to save life (Exod. 1:19f.; 1 Sam. 16:1-3; 2 Kings 6:14-20). Deceit in this area, of course, could provoke lawsuits. Therefore it is best for a physician to avoid examining a fetus for potential birth defects unless the mother agrees in advance not to abort the child.

D. CONFIDENTIALITY

Should a physician inform a girl's parents that she is pregnant, has a venereal disease, or uses contraceptives? Should a psychiatrist tell the police (or the intended victim or both) that his patient intends to kill someone? Should he tell a patient's fiancée that the

33. No physical condition determines or forces anyone to commit sin. If it did, that condition would be an *excuse* for sin, and Scripture allows no such excuses. It is clear, however, that physical conditions (among other circumstances) influence the particular range of *temptations* that an individual faces. The fact that one is wealthy may tempt one to set his heart on riches (1 Tim. 6:17). A person with a severe handicap may be tempted toward bitterness or over-dependence on others. A person suffering pain may be tempted to speak rudely to those he finds annoying. So I do consider it possible that genetic or other physical factors may be genuine causes for moral concern. I would not rule out the possibility that there are genetic factors that predispose people to the temptations of, for example, alcoholism and homosexuality.

34. See Beauchamp and Childress, 208; also V. Elving Anderson, "Biological Engineering and the Future of Man," in Carl F. H. Henry, 158f.

patient is a homosexual? In a word, Yes. A pregnant or promiscuous teenager, for example, needs help, and her parents are responsible for giving her that help. Although a physician should respect the authority and unity of the family, if there is reason to believe that her parents would abuse her if told the truth, then they are "incompetent," and she should be placed in other hands. Otherwise, the parents should be given the benefit of the doubt and the help of their physician.

Scripture warrants confidentiality up to a point. It condemns gossip, which includes discussing someone's problems with people who cannot help (Prov. 18:8; 26:17ff.), talkativeness (Prov. 10:19; 29:20; Eccl. 5:2ff.; 10:14), and, generally, revealing secrets (Prov. 11:13). But according to Scripture, confidentiality is not an absolute. Sometimes what we hear *should* be repeated. If I hear that someone has something against me, I must go to that person and ask him about it (Matt. 5:23f.). When asked to give legal testimony, I must tell the truth; I must reveal as much as is relevant to a just disposition of the case (Exod. 23:2f.). There is a time for silence and a time for speech (Eccl. 3:7), and the latter is the time when our words should edify, should serve a useful purpose in God's economy (1 Cor. 14:26; Eph. 4:29). All that I said earlier about our obligation to do good applies here, for words are one tool for doing good. Therefore patients should be told that though the physician is not a gossip, he cannot give an unequivocal promise of confidentiality. He will keep confidences only as far as his conscience permits. Scripture warns us against rash oaths, and an unconditional promise of confidentiality cannot help but be rash, since we never know when we will be obligated to repeat something we have been told.

One argument in *favor* of absolute confidentiality is that without it, fewer people will seek medical counsel, resulting in a greater net amount of harm.[35] But that is a utilitarian argument and a somewhat speculative one at best. In any case, God's law, which obligates us to do good, must take precedence over utilitarian arguments. It would be unfortunate if some people rejected medical treatment out of fear that their sin might be exposed. But for some

35. Mentioned, but not endorsed, by Beauchamp and Childress, 4.

people, that may be part of the price they must pay for disobeying God's law.

To say that is to contradict the current legal trends.[36] We should not disobey the law unless conscience (and therefore God's law) requires it. To minimize conflicts over confidentiality, before examining and treating a patient with a medically sensitive problem, a physician should require the patient to agree to allow him to follow biblical principles of confidentiality.

E. JUSTICE

How is health care to be distributed throughout society? Does each person have a right to "equal treatment"? If so, what would that mean? If not, who takes precedence over whom?

Such questions are often described as questions about justice. Justice declares that the benefits and burdens of life should be distributed according to desert. But how do we tell who deserves what? Applying different principles yields different results. Should distribution be according to equality, to need, to effort, to social contribution, to merit, or to some combination of these?[37] If we decide to distribute according to "need," for example, we must still determine what needs are genuine and what needs are the most important.

I believe that different principles take precedence in different areas of life. Surely merit and achievement should play the major role in qualifying persons for jobs, offices, and honors in society. Not everyone can be president of General Motors or receive the Nobel Peace Prize, so it would be absurd to consider that such honors be distributed on the basis of equality or of need. Not even communist societies claim equality at that level.

With regard to medical care, then, I trust that without fear of being called a socialist I can say that the chief criterion is need.

36. See Payne's important observations in this regard, 119f. In this book I am not trying to reflect on the legal aspects of medical ethics, a dimension of the topic on which I am largely ignorant. Rather, I am speaking ethically; I am speaking about what the laws *should* be and of how we *should* behave, regardless of what civil law may require.

37. Beauchamp and Childress, 172ff.

Our earlier discussions of beneficence, the Good Samaritan, and related topics should make that obvious. The point is virtually tautological, for the primary purpose of medicine is to help people who have certain kinds of needs, to reduce inequalities caused by disease or injury. We see someone bleeding on the road, and we help him the best we can; that's the essence of it. From this truism one might deduce that we should seek to minimize inequalities of access to medical care. The man bleeding on the road cannot walk into the hospital as others can. He needs someone to carry him, to help him, to get him walking again. Often there are *economic* barriers to healing that must be overcome. The Good Samaritan left *money* to pay for rest and treatment. If healing requires blood, then blood should be provided; if a kidney, then a kidney should be found; if money, then money should be given. Whatever is needed should be supplied.

Who is responsible for bearing those burdens and expenses? Initially the patient is, for Scripture teaches that we are responsible for ourselves. But when we can no longer bear our burdens and expenses, God has provided us with our family. And when our family fails, God has provided us with the church. I do not believe, however, that Scripture teaches that the state has a role in welfare (my capitalist credentials remain untarnished!).

When someone is bleeding by the side of the road, without money and without obvious family or church connections, the potential healer may have to sacrifice not only time and skill but also financial resources, as the Good Samaritan did. In the Old Testament, God's people were told not to charge interest on loans to their needy neighbors (Exod. 22:25ff.); and in the New Testament, they shared their goods freely. Spontaneous response to need, not letting the left hand know what the right hand does, is something God honors.

There are limits to generosity, of course. Scripture does not require that anyone become bankrupt through unreimbursed charity. There is always an element of free choice where charity is concerned. The Old Testament mandates openhandedness toward the poor in a general way (Deut. 15:7-11) and forbids interest on charity loans, but it does not require anyone to impoverish himself by lending money he needs for essentials. The early Christians were not *required* to sell all their houses and lands (Acts 5:4). Paul makes it clear that the offering for the poor is not intended to impoverish anyone; rather, the burden is to be shared equally (Acts 8:13-15). Making an extraordinary sacrifice may often (when not foolish!) be a praiseworthy action, and thus an "obligation" in the sense of chapter 1, B, 9, d, above, but, as I discussed in that section, such sacrifices are not equally binding on all.

Surely, then, Christian physicians and hospitals are not required to bear, overall, a disproportionate share of the burden. They may, like the Samaritan, be called upon to make the initial outlay of funds, but they should be reimbursed by the community so that the sacrifice is equalized. In the Old Testament, welfare was financed through the tithes of all the people; in the New Testament (in addition to the tithe, I believe), the poor were fed through general appeals for free-will offerings.

Administration of such funds in Scripture is the responsibility of the church, not the state. What if the patient belongs to a different denomination from his healers or to no church at all? The Good Samaritan story suggests that God's people should give aid to the sick and injured without asking questions about religious affiliation.

I believe that if Christians were to tithe their incomes and if Christian churches would unite, there would be sufficient funds available to meet the needs we have been discussing. (Church unity is important because denominational barriers hinder communication and free sharing within the Christian community. If the church were one, a group of Christians with a disproportionate burden could readily appeal to other groups with the firm expectation of help.) Since this is God's way of meeting this need, He will certainly provide.

Another especially difficult question in this context is that of "microallocation," the question of "which persons will receive some scarce preventive or therapeutic procedure."[38] Various criteria have been proposed for choosing among patients for such procedures: need, geographical proximity, constituency factors (e.g.,

38. Ibid., 192. The question of "macroallocation"—the priorities for social investment in various medical procedures—is discussed briefly under chapter 1, C, 8.

veterans have precedence at V.A. hospitals), prospect of success, progress of science (i.e., will use of a new technique on person A advance our scientific understanding more than the use of it on person B?), social worth, random selection, and queuing (first come, first served). And in some cases, the ability to pay is also an operative criterion, whether or not it is acknowledged as such.

How, then, can we best microallocate scarce medical resources? Here are some suggestions.

a. Just as the chief criterion for administering medical care is need, I believe that need is the chief criterion for microallocating medical resources. Once again, the model of the Good Samaritan is fundamental: When we see someone in need, we should help without asking whether he "truly" qualifies as a neighbor, that is, without asking questions about his wealth, social utility, religious belief, and so forth.

b. At times, however, we learn about many needs simultaneously and cannot handle them all at once. The second criterion—choose a system of priorities that maximizes the help given—is closely related to the first. Several principles can help us apply this criterion. (i) Geographical factors will sometimes play a role. We can usually meet more needs if we focus on those closest to us, rather than spending valuable time in travel and transport. (ii) In some situations the concept of "social worth" should be taken into account. In case of a mass disaster, for example, doctors and nurses should be given priority so that they can help others.[39] It is important to note that we are not making broad judgments about who is more valuable to society as a whole; we are only determining who will make the greatest contribution to the medical needs before us. (iii) "Prospect of success" is another important criterion in this context. Scarce medical resources should be spent on those who can best use them, which means that they certainly should not be used merely to prolong the process of dying (see c, below.) (iv) "Progress of science" is a criterion that will rarely be relevant, but there may be occasions to use it. Imagine that there is an epidemic that could be relieved by an experimental vaccine but that the government is

39. Similarly, "sailors on an overloaded craft in a storm" (Ibid., 197) should be given priority so that they can help save the ship.

unwilling to approve the vaccine until tests are made on persons within a certain category. In that case, the "progress of science" criterion becomes an application of the "need" criterion, for such research is necessary to maximize help.

c. Following those considerations, it seems to me that queuing or, if it is impossible to determine the order in which needs were manifested, random selection should be the determining factor. And that is a way of reiterating our emphasis on perceived need as the chief criterion for microallocating medical resources. It is also a way of making a generally negative judgment against other criteria that might be suggested. For example, (i) "ability to pay" should not be a consideration. Funding of medical care should in all cases rest first on the patient himself, then his family, then the church, as discussed earlier in this section. The physician or hospital may have to make the initial outlay of funds, but they should be reimbursed by those who bear the responsibility. Nor should (ii) "general considerations of social worth" beyond the applications discussed above under *b*, *(ii)* be a consideration: How can we refuse to help someone before us in order to help someone "more important"? James 2:1-7 suggests some analogies at this point, and the biblical teaching that the poor are not to be exploited in legal matters also is relevant.[40] Making broad judgments about the worth of people to society in general is unscriptural in my view, though it is sometimes recommended by medical ethicists. All lives are precious because they bear God's image. And in the church, each member depends on every other member (1 Cor. 12). Finally, (iii) "constituency factors" should not be a criterion of selection; someone outside of the constituency should not *a priori* be denied treatment. Once again the model of the Good Samaritan refutes such thinking. Of course it is natural that veterans will predominate at veterans hospitals, and Catholics at Catholic hospitals, and so forth. And evangelical Christians will normally turn to other Evangelicals for help. The church is a kind of extension of the family, and

40. I agree with Beauchamp and Childress that "perhaps the president of the country in wartime would be given priority" (198). They add, however, "But in few cases would particular patients be truly indispensable to society." All nations (including Old Testament Israel) took special precautions to protect their heads of state.

the family must care for its own. But there is no justification for rejecting someone simply because he does not belong to our group. The proper balance is summed up in the following verse: "Therefore, as we have opportunity, let us do good to all people, especially to those who belong to the family of believers" (Gal. 6:10).

3

THE SITUATIONAL PERSPECTIVE: SOME PROBLEM AREAS

In this section we will discuss several types of medical situations that give rise to especially difficult ethical questions. One problem I shall not discuss here is the problem of abortion, about which I have written extensively elsewhere. I am including as Appendix B a denominational statement on abortion of which I was the chief author.[1] Nor will I discuss questions surrounding genetic engineering or the "new reproduction" (*in vitro* fertilization, surrogate parenting, etc.), which may, however, find their way into a future book. And, important though it is today, I must set aside for now the difficult questions surrounding AIDS, though my discussions of confidentiality and of terminal illness are certainly applicable to

1. See also my article in Richard Ganz, ed., *Thou Shalt Not Kill* (New Rochelle, N.Y.: Arlington House, 1978), 43-75, and references to abortion earlier in this book, especially under chapter 2, A.

that disease. New information and new claims about AIDS appear nearly every week, and I am not now in a position to sort out that information and those claims. In general, I believe that AIDS should be handled more as a communicable disease and less as a civil rights issue; I am appalled at the restrictions many states have placed on the communication of information concerning AIDS carriers to health authorities.

But there are other problems that will keep us busy enough in this section.

A. MEDICAL RESEARCH

Research on human subjects is especially problematic because the medical interests of the participating physicians are broader than their concern for the patients' (and/or subjects') well-being.[2] For that and other reasons, many criteria have been suggested for guiding medical research on human beings. Among these criteria are the following:

a. Research should be conducted by qualified persons.

b. Human subjects should be used only when necessary and only after sufficient laboratory and animal experimentation.

c. The perceived benefits should outweigh the possible risks.

d. Informed consent should be obtained from subjects.

e. Rigorous safeguards should be taken to prevent harm; unintended psychological alteration should especially be guarded against.

f. There should be a morally important reason for the research.

g. There should be a reasonable prospect that the experiment will achieve its goal.

2. Tom L. Beauchamp and James F. Childress, *Principles of Biomedical Ethics* (New York: Oxford University Press, 1979), 80, 221.

h. There should not be a disproportionate number of power-less, poor, weak, imprisoned, or institutionalized subjects so that the burdens of the research may be fairly distributed throughout society.[3]

Those criteria are good rules of thumb and good safeguards against abusing human subjects in medical research. In cases such as a plague of epidemic proportions, however, I think that all of them except f could be relaxed to some extent without compromising any biblical principles. When the goal of research is healing, I believe that the model of the Good Samaritan indicates that the research should be completed quickly for the sake of those who need the treatment that is under investigation. Sometimes that consideration will militate against multiplying safeguards or against rigidly complying with them or both.

Randomized clinical trials, in which persons are randomly assigned to treatment categories where they receive an experimental treatment or a placebo, present a particular set of problems.[4] Hanley Abramson notes:

This procedure was followed in the 1954 field trials of the Salk polio vaccine, except, of course, that parents had to give the consent for their children. It is obvious that a certain number of children contracted polio and died as a result of receiving the placebo instead of the vaccine.[5]

He adds, however, that "the risk to the control group was not greater than before the trial of the vaccine, which had potential hazards of its own; and the controlled trial was the only way to determine whether or not the vaccine was effective."

Beauchamp and Childress stipulate several "necessary conditions" that must be met to justify randomized clinical trials. They

3. See Lewis P. Bird, "Dilemmas in Biomedical Ethics," in Carl F. H. Henry, ed., *Horizons of Science* (San Francisco: Harper and Row, 1978), 145; also James F. Childress, *Priorities in Biomedical Ethics* (Philadelphia: Westminster Press, 1981), 55-58.

4. Beauchamp and Childress (74) define randomized clinical trials as "random assignment to treatment categories where there are alternative treatments—in which some patients receive placebos or an experimental therapy, e.g., a drug, while other patients receive a standard or alternative therapy."

5. "Ethical Concerns in Drug Research," in Charles Hatfield, ed., *The Scientist and Ethical Decision* (Downers Grove, Ill.: Inter-Varsity Press, 1973), 54f.

argue that these conditions are necessary but not sufficient since other conditions may have to be met in particular cases. Here are their conditions.

(i) There is no satisfactory alternative methodology which avoids the problem of withholding information. (ii) The subjects are informed that they are involved in a randomized clinical trial and might be receiving a placebo or a nonvalidated therapy. (iii) The research is well designed, including provisions for the evaluation of the alternative therapies. (iv) All therapies to be included have no substantial disparity in their prior probabilities of benefit. (v) Risks to patients are fully detailed prior to their consent and are minimal (e.g., not beyond the risk involved in a standard physical examination) if there is a risk that cannot be divulged. (vi) Consent safeguards, such as a surrogate consent system, have been put in place wherever appropriate.[6]

I have several reservations about *(iv)*. If administering placebos can be justified in this context, why can't we justify administering to one group a treatment that is initially thought to have less probability of effectiveness? Such a procedure might provide more protection to the patients than the placebo alternative, and it could provide useful information for the researchers. Certainly, however, the other five safeguards (and even *(iv)* in many cases) have a *prima facie* validity. Granting once again the need for flexibility in emergency situations, it is certainly desirable to maximize patient information and choice and to minimize risk.

Beauchamp and Childress raise questions about the necessity of the widespread use of randomized clinical trials. "The increased probability of their results is only a matter of degree, and there may be reasons for preferring a less conclusive method if it would more fully respect our duties to current patients."[7] But there are future patients to consider, so some weighing and balancing is in order.

Additional questions about the ethical propriety of medical research on human beings concern the participation of persons

---

6. Beauchamp and Childress, 75.
7. Ibid., 222.

from the following groups: children, the unborn, the mentally disabled, prisoners, and other institutionalized persons. The logic of informed consent dictates that adult subjects normally should be preferred to children and that older children should be preferred to younger ones. Beauchamp and Childress also point out that it is easier to avoid doing harm to adults than to children because adults are able to communicate better than children.[8] There are cases (such as studies of diseases largely limited to childhood or studies of the effects of any disease upon children) where the participation of children in research is essential. But in these cases, informed parental consent and risk safeguards are especially important. And in such cases, unborn children, including fertilized eggs *in vitro*, have the same rights as children already born. If anything, such subjects should be treated all the more carefully since they are the *youngest* and the least able to give informed consent and to communicate need.[9]

Caution, of course, must be employed in the use of institutionalized subjects, but I do believe that in many cases adequate safeguards are possible. Committees of wise people[10] from outside the institution can judge whether improper pressure has been placed upon the subjects to participate.

The mentally disabled present a special problem since they are often incompetent to give consent and have no adequate proxies to give that consent. Studies of such persons and of their conditions are necessary, however, to help advance the treatment of mental disabilities. In these cases the physician (perhaps with the assistance of review committees)[11] must take responsibility for the interests of his patient. Should the mentally disabled be used in experiments unrelated to mental disabilities? As a rule, I do not believe they should be, unless the patient has some other problem the study of which would be useful and would not put him at any greater risk.[12]

8. Ibid., 179.
9. See Appendix B.
10. For the importance of church participation in such a process, see chapter 2, C.
11. See the immediately preceding note.
12. See the discussion in Beauchamp and Childress, 182f.

In biblical terms, medical research should be regarded as part of the process of healing people. As such, it has the same biblical mandate as medical treatment itself. The difference between researched and unresearched medical treatments is the difference (other things being equal) between acting with the wisdom gained through research and not acting with such wisdom. Thus though safeguards are important, clinical trials are not inherently suspect from an ethical point of view; and their results, though subject to human fallibility, should be received with thanksgiving to God.

B. CRITERIA OF DEATH

We now turn to the issues surrounding death and dying. Scripture does not formally define physical death but assumes that we understand what it is. Scripture speaks about death in the everyday language of ordinary experience, not in technical terms. Clearly, however, Scripture does recognize a point at which efforts to save a person's life, even by prayer, are to be abandoned (see especially 2 Sam. 12:19-23). At that point the proper treatment of the body is burial (Gen. 23:4ff.; Deut. 21:23; John 19:40). If there is any criterion[13] of death noted in the scriptural accounts, it would be cessation of breathing,[14] though Scripture does not present this as a technical criterion but simply as a matter of empirical observation.

Other empirical signs of death can be enumerated: cessation of heartbeat,[15] reflexes, body heat, flexibility, and cell growth and the eventual putrefaction and decomposition of the body. More recent studies have added to this list the cessation of brain activity.

The heart, lungs, and brain seem to be the major organs governing the principal signs of life. They are, respectively, the sources of

13. I prefer to speak of "criterion" rather than of "definition." I'm not sure that a "definition" (at least of a technical and nontheological sort) of death is possible. In any case, I doubt if any of the proposed criteria of death really constitute definitions in any significant sense. They seem, rather, to be symptoms of that separation of soul from body that Scripture identifies as death.

14. Josh. 11:11ff.; 1 Kings 15:29; 17:17; Job 27:3; Ps. 104:29; Isa. 2:22; cf. Gen. 2:7; 6:17; 7:15, 22; Ezek. 37:5ff.; Acts 17:25.

15. The centrality of the heart to man's physical life is perhaps noted in Scripture by the metaphorical use of "heart" to designate the most basic dimension of a person's nature (Prov. 4:23, etc.).

circulation, breathing, and direction. But any of these may lose its function for a period of time and later be restored. Circulation and breathing, indeed, can be maintained by artificial means, and it is not impossible to imagine a time when some (perhaps minimal) brain activity also may be maintained artificially.

The heart, lungs, and brain are mutually dependent. The brain requires oxygen and blood; lung operation requires blood and brain-direction; heartbeat requires oxygen from the lungs, which in turn are dependent on brain-function. Therefore, when one function is lost for a long enough time, the others will be lost as well. But, again, complications arise when functions otherwise lacking are maintained artificially. One cannot really tell if a patient has lost lung and heart function unless the patient is removed from the artificial life-support system, though to do that to a living but sick patient might be dangerous.

Increasingly, then, the tendency is to use brain-death as a criterion of death. Because in many cases the artificial maintenance of circulation and respiration makes it difficult to use the cessation of those functions as criteria for death, loss of brain function is the remaining plausible alternative. This alternative has become even more attractive as organ-transplant technology has developed. If people can be declared dead while still on heart/lung machines, their organs can more easily be "harvested" for transplant purposes.

The President's Commission for the Study of Ethical Problems in Medicine and Biomedical and Behavioral Research (1981) defined death as *either* the (1) irreversible cessation of circulatory and respiratory functions *or* the (2) irreversible cessation of all functions of the entire brain, including the brain stem.[16] This language is incorporated into the Uniform Determination of Death Act (UDDA), a piece of model legislation that has been enacted (often with some modification) by over thirty state legislatures.

One wonders, though, what would happen if a technology were developed to maintain brain function artificially. For a patient on artificial heart, lung, *and brain* support, how would the physician determine death? Indeed, what if all the signs of death (including

16. Quoted in Franklin Payne, *Biblical/Medical Ethics* (Milford, Mich.: Mott Media, 1985), 205.

lowered body temperature, etc.) could be artificially postponed? How would the physician know when or if death had occurred? How, indeed, would he know when, in effect, the living person had become a robot? This observation indicates that loss of brain function is not a criterion inherently superior to the others; it just happens to be more convenient given our present state of technology. If the brain and heart but not the lungs could be sustained artificially, then "lung-death" would be the prevalent criterion and the one under discussion in medical ethics.

The term "irreversible" in the commission's formulation also is important and indicates a certain looseness in the definition, for it is sometimes difficult to determine when loss of function is irreversible. Irreversibility, too, is technology-dependent: medical science must seek ways in which to reverse losses of function that until now have been irreversible. Still, it is necessary for physicians to make some judgment concerning what, at a particular point in history, they can or cannot do to restore a patient. Doubtless some people were buried in biblical times who could have been resuscitated by twentieth-century technology. Those who did the burying, however, were not guilty of sin, since God did not expect them to understand what medical technology would be capable of thousands of years in the future.

The phrase "entire brain" in the commission's formulation counters the suggestion that loss of neocortical function (which governs speech, reason, and "higher human capacities") is sufficient to warrant a declaration of death. Suggesting that loss of neocortical function is a sufficient criterion of death reflects an unbiblical attempt to define humanity or personality according to the "higher" functions and thus to declare one who has lost those functions as less than human. Against this sort of proposal, see chapter 2, A, above. The commission's formulation rightly rejects defining death as a loss of neocortical function. Questions have been raised, however, about how the UDDA will be used in practice. The explanatory booklet of the president's commission opens the door wider to more liberal practices in the determination of death than a literal reading of its recommendations might suggest. On this discussion, see my Appendix A.

Appendix A also investigates the propriety of a "functional" definition of death (in this context, a definition in terms of brain, heart, and lung functions) as opposed to "substantial" definitions (which require the "destruction" of organs). Anticipating my treatment of these issues, I would say here that a total loss of function is what we *mean* by "destruction" in most cases, so that the two sorts of definitions are basically equivalent. But functional definitions *sound* less strict and thus can be used to justify what to some of us seem like premature declarations of death.

My own conclusion is that we should not declare someone dead until we can conclude that heart, lungs, and brain have *all* irreversibly ceased to function. Perhaps we should also postpone the declaration until other processes associated with death (kidney failure, lowered body temperature, etc.) have at least begun to manifest themselves. That last point notwithstanding, the UDDA, even on its most literal reading, is too liberal: it defines two different sets of conditions as separate, independent criteria of death. Thus, for example, using the UDDA definition of death, someone who is "brain dead" but who has a good heart and lungs may be declared dead, though in some cases such persons have been resuscitated. Therefore it is better to define death as the irreversible loss of heart, lung, and brain function—to make each a necessary criterion and all three together the sufficient criteria for declaring someone to be dead. This will mean, of course, that when someone is "brain dead" but supported by ventilators and so forth, he may have to be removed from those machines to determine whether he has died, or, perhaps, if he is still alive, to "let him die" (see C, 3 below).

In any case physicians must think long and hard before declaring someone to have "irreversibly" lost *all* brain function from "all parts of the brain, even the brain stem." Surely conventional methods, such as the EEG, do not justify such extreme conclusions. Is it really possible to conclude such a thing in the absence of the deterioration of other organs? Thus even the UDDA concept of brain-death, if taken seriously (and some have charged that it is not to be taken seriously, see Appendix A) requires more than brain-data for its proper implementation. Thus a definition of death that is more strict than "brain-death" alone is needed, though certainly the loss of brain function is one significant indicator among others.

Without a strict criterion of death, it is difficult to guard against abuses, such as hastening a declaration of death to obtain organs for transplant. Ideally, the physician(s) responsible for determining the death of a patient should have no interest in the transplant process, though practically it is hard to avoid a conflict of interest in that situation. Second and third opinions, review committees, and so forth are of some use, but multiple appeals can take up valuable time. These issues must be resolved case by case. But if the transplant process is not to become an excuse for another holocaust (like the abortion holocaust), stricter controls than those presently in common use are needed.

Recent stories about the use of fetuses and anencephalic children for transplants, and of fetal tissue to treat Parkinson's disease, are a particular case in point.[17] There is no problem if the child-donor has died of irreversible natural causes, as was evidently the case in the use of fetal tissue for Parkinson's patients reported by *Time*. But clearly (granted the argument of Appendix B) it would be wrong to abort a fetus to supply transplant materials. The wrong here is in the abortion itself, rather than the use of the fetus for transplants; but if the latter becomes widespread practice it could be used as another justification for abortion, which would be most unfortunate. Rumors that some women are considering becoming pregnant with the express purpose of aborting the fetus and donating it (even, perhaps, selling it!) for medical treatment are most disturbing.

We should, therefore, employ a strict definition of death for both born and unborn patients; and we should never *put* anyone to death, born or unborn.[18]

C. SOME IMPORTANT DISTINCTIONS

As we saw in the last section, clarity of thought in medical ethics often requires the careful use of terms. The following distinctions

17. See "A Balancing Act of Life and Death," *Time* (Feb. 1, 1988): 49. For a report citing various Christian responses, see Arthur H. Matthews, "Ethicists Concerned After Quintuplets' Birth, Tissue Use in Mexico," *World* (Jan. 25, 1988): 4-5.
18. Is it ever justified to postpone by artificial means an inevitable death to preserve organs for transplants? I would say yes, within limits: see C, 3 below.

are frequently discussed, especially in the areas of death and terminal illness.

1. CONDITIONS OF PATIENTS

a. In the previous section we discussed the concept of death, that is, what it means to say that a patient has *died*. It is important that this condition be distinguished from the next.

b. The *dying* patient. Dying is not, of course, the same as death. One who is dying is still alive, and our responsibility to that patient is not to bury him but to give care.

What does it mean for a patient to be dying? Sometimes we use the word to describe a patient who would die if he were given no medical care at all, as in the phrase "dying by the side of the road." Patients who are dying in that sense often can be restored to good health. The word "dying" also may be used of those who are under medical care but for whom that medical care is not successful, and that is how I will use the term.

How do we tell when a patient is dying? I cannot draw a sharp line between dying and nondying patients; physicians must do their best to make an accurate judgment in each case. In general, when the physician knows that no further treatment will prevent imminent death (as understood under B), he knows that the patient is dying. Under "preventing death," I would not include the mere preservation of functions through artificial life support, for that is, to some extent, compatible with death as we have described it.

Death is, of course, the "last enemy" (1 Cor. 15:26), but it is not on that account always to be resisted (Gen. 49:33; Matt. 27:50; Acts 21:13; 25:11; Rom. 14:7f.; Phil. 1:21). God's people can accept death because they look forward to the certainty of immediate fellowship with God and the future resurrection of the body. They are not suicidal, but when it is evident that their life is at an end, they do not desperately, against all natural probability, seek its prolongation.

How should we care for dying patients? Some treatments, of course, should be discontinued. When a physician is convinced that certain treatments intended to prevent death cannot succeed, he should stop them. But treatment intended to maintain the patient's comfort and normal functioning must continue. Nourishment, water, oxygen, and shelter are essential, even when they must be administered "artificially."[19] Similarly, treatment that is intended to prevent death from a condition other than that from which the patient is dying must continue; until the patient is *dead*, he is a living human being, a proper object of the love, care, and prayers of others.

Hospice care and (even better) home care often provide better environments than hospitals for patients that are dying. Unless there are complications (such as secondary conditions that require medical treatment that otherwise would leave the patient in pain), those alternatives deserve consideration.[20]

c. The *comatose* patient. It is important to distinguish coma from death and from dying. Comatose patients are not dead, and often they are not even dying. People can live for many years in a comatose condition. Karen Ann Quinlan lived many years in a comatose state after she was removed, by legal action, from a respirator. For most of that period she was neither dead nor dying. There have been many "surprising" recoveries of patients who have been comatose for years.

Comatose patients should receive all the care due to dying patients (above, *b*), as well as whatever treatments may reasonably be expected to revive them from their comas. In many cases, however, such treatments may not exist, and in such cases treatment of the comatose will be similar to treatment of the dying.

d. The *terminal* patient. Terminal patients are those who have illnesses or injuries from which, according to the best medical judgment, they will *eventually* die. These patients, too, however, must be distinguished from patients who either are dead or dying. Terminal patients may live for many years. And unlike the comatose, they may live active lives during those years. Terminal patients should be treated medically to maintain their normal functioning as much as possible (as with *b*). And normally they should be given treatment to prolong their lives until it is evident that dying has

---

19. One of my medical correspondents asks, "*How* artificial?" noting that respirators, for example, are artificial. I would say that respirators and other "artificial" means should be used to maintain comfort and function unless these themselves become barriers to "letting die," when "letting die" is justified. See below, C, 3.

20. See Payne, 191f.

begun or that death has occurred. I do not believe, however, that in choosing among treatments it is always necessary to choose the one that prolongs life the longest. In view of the Scripture texts cited under *b* above (also chapter 1, C, 3, *b*), I believe that in some cases a Christian may responsibly refuse treatment or choose a treatment that will extend his life for a shorter period of time than other treatments (see below, 2 and 3). And those who make proxy consent for incompetent patients, such as Joseph Saikewicz (the case with which I opened this book), may responsibly make the same sort of decision.

e. The *handicapped* patient. Like comatose patients, some handicapped patients may be nonsapient, that is, incapable of significant communication and interaction with others. But they are not on that account to be abandoned. They may be neither dead nor dying nor comatose nor even terminally ill. They should be treated for their condition as much as possible, provided with normal life support, and given whatever is necessary and possible to make their lives as normal as can be.

The distinctions we have just made are often ignored, at least in popular discussions of medical ethics. Terms such as "vegetable" and "bodies without persons" greatly inhibit clarity. Comatose, terminal, or severely handicapped patients are often described as if they were dying or already dead. The issues are difficult enough without that sort of obfuscation.

2. ORDINARY AND EXTRAORDINARY CARE

Gerald Kelly, S.J., formulates the distinction between ordinary and extraordinary care as follows:

> Ordinary means are all medicines, treatments, and operations, which offer a reasonable hope of benefit and which can be obtained and used without excessive expense, pain or other inconvenience. Extraordinary means are all medicines, treatments, and operations, which cannot be obtained or used without excessive expense, pain, or other inconvenience, or which, if used, would not offer a reasonable hope of benefit.[21]

21. Quoted in Beauchamp and Childress, 118. The reference is to Kelly, "The Duty to Preserve Life," *Theological Studies* (Dec. 1951): 550.

It is evident that this definition is less than precise. There is often room for debate over what is or is not a "reasonable hope of benefit" and over what is or is not "excessive." Often such debates are resolved by custom: "ordinary care" is what is customarily performed, "extraordinary" is anything beyond that. Simply to accept custom as self-validating, however, is to abdicate our responsibility to make moral assessments.

Beauchamp and Childress prefer to distinguish (morally) "obligatory" means of treatment from "optional" means of treatment. Treatment is optional if it is not likely to be beneficial or if it imposes burdens that outweigh the benefits offered.[22] But they recognize that the second criterion is difficult to apply. In the absence of communication, thought, and consciousness, is life itself a benefit? What about children with Tay-Sachs? With spina bifida? With Down's syndrome? What of the *economic* burdens to the patient or to his family?

According to Scripture, life *is* a benefit. Not only is it sacred and not to be taken by man (Gen. 9:6; Exod. 20:13) but length of days is a covenantal blessing (Prov. 3:2). We have no right to say that a handicapped person's life is not worth living. Even the most severe suffering does not render our lives valueless (see Rom. 8:18; 2 Cor. 4:11-18 and chapters 11 and 12; Heb. 11).

Still, as indicated in the passages cited in *1, b* above (and chapter 1, C, 3, b), physical longevity is not the supreme value that is to be increased at all other costs. One may accept death simply because it is inevitable or by risking it for God or for other people. Therefore an individual may responsibly reject a treatment out of unwillingness to burden his family, even in an economic sense.

What of those who are incapable of giving informed consent? I think that proxies, as in the Saikewicz case, are competent to make determinations that are in the best interest of the patient. Thus I believe that the court was right to rule that chemotherapy would impose suffering on Saikewicz that would be disproportionate to the value of (possibly) adding a few days to his life. It would not have been right, however, for anyone to *require* that he act self-sacrificially for the sake of others. Although a parent may find it a

---

22. Beauchamp and Childress, 119ff.

great economic burden to maintain a severely handicapped child, he
has no right to refuse treatment merely to ease his own burdens.[23]

3. KILLING AND LETTING DIE

This distinction is sometimes criticized as making no moral difference,[24] and in some cases it does not. If my uncle is dying and I
withhold his heart medicine without which he will die, I am, in
one sense, "letting die," not "killing." But surely in that situation I
am as responsible for his death as if I had shot him through the
heart. There are, however, many cases where the distinction *does*
make a difference. For example, there are many in the world who
are dying and whom we are not presently seeking to help. In one
sense we are "letting them die," but few would argue that we are
their murderers.[25] Consider another example. Several swimmers
are drowning, and we can only rescue one. If we do so, then we are
"letting (the others) die." But no one would argue that that decision is wrong in itself. It would, however, clearly be wrong for us to
shoot the other swimmers to death!

Thus "letting die" is not *always* morally justified, though *sometimes* it is. When may we let a patient die? In general I would say
that we may let a patient die when we lack, in some way, the resources to save his life, whether those resources be time, technology, or skill. When a person is under medical care, we may let him
die (in terms of our earlier definition) when he is "dying."

This principle does *not* justify withholding treatment from "bodies without persons," "people without a personal future," or "people with horrible burdens."[26] Persons such as these are in the image of God (above, chapter 2, A) and deserve care as much as anyone else. I am not saying that such persons, however, must always
be given maximal care. Allow me to reiterate. (a) A patient but not

23. As I said earlier, however, the Christian community has a responsibility to
equalize such burdens.
24. See the discussion of Rachels's argument in Beauchamp and Childress, 107ff.
25. There is, of course, room for discussion about our duty toward those who
are, for example, starving in Africa.
26. As Lewis Smedes maintains in *Mere Morality* (Grand Rapids: Wm. B. Eerdmans Publishing Co., 1983), 148-51.

his proxies may refuse maximal treatment to spare others terrible burdens and expenses—a self-sacrificial motive. (b) A patient or proxy may determine, as in the Saikewicz case, to use a treatment that minimizes suffering rather than one which maximizes length of life. These patients, generally, are not dying when the decisions in question are made. At that time, then, these are not cases of "letting die" (in terms of our definition), though they become so once the patient actually begins to die.

Certainly none of these observations justifies killing handicapped infants by starvation and dehydration, for example, as in the famous "Baby Doe" case.[27] This sort of thing is as culpable as active killing.

In the cases of just war, capital punishment, and self-defense, killing is justified.[28] Rarely, if ever, however, do those exceptions to the prohibition against taking life justify killing a medical patient in the process of treatment. Therefore we can say that for practical purposes killing is never justified as a part of medical care, though "letting die" sometimes is.

"Mercy killing," or killing to relieve suffering, is sometimes defended by ethicists. Today that is the usual meaning of *euthanasia*, though originally the term referred to the giving of comfort to dying patients. "Mercy-killing" is sometimes described as *active* euthanasia and distinguished from "letting die" or *passive* euthanasia. The ethically relevant differences between killing and letting die, however, are so great that I prefer not to make them members of one terminological species. Terminology such as "active euthanasia" and "passive euthanasia" encourages illegitimate moral equations between the two; those who in some cases are reconciled to "passive euthanasia" may find it too easy to accept "active euthanasia" as well.

27. This is discussed in many places. See, e.g., Payne, 1ff., 197. That a number of families pleaded to adopt this Down's syndrome child made the procedure all the more appalling.
28. Of course, this position is controversial, but I don't think it is useful to discuss these matters in detail, since I have little to add to the great volume of literature on these subjects. My position is the traditional Reformed view, which is based on passages such as Genesis 9:6; Exodus 22:2; Deuteronomy 20; Acts 25:11; and Romans 13:1-5.

Scripture always presents mercy killing negatively.[29] Consider the following. (a) People in the Bible who either killed themselves or who sought to have themselves killed to avoid suffering are always seen as disobedient (Judges 9:54-57; 1 Sam. 31:3-6; 2 Sam. 1:9-16; 17:23; 1 Kings 16:15-19; Matt. 27:5; Acts 1:18). (b) The command against murder includes murder of the self; suicide contradicts the legitimate self-love that Scripture assumes and commends (Matt. 22:39; Eph. 5:28). (c) Suffering does not render a life meaningless or valueless (Rom. 8:18; 2 Cor. 4:11-18 and chapters 11 and 12). (d) Our lives are not our own; they are not at our own disposal (1 Cor. 6:19f.; 7:4). So "letting die" is sometimes justified, though "killing" never is. Is "letting die" ever an *obligation*? Are there cases where we *must* let someone die?

This question is important today because of transplant technology. Organs generally lose their value for transplant purposes if they are "harvested" too long after the death of the donor. Thus physicians are sometimes tempted to keep a patient on artificial life support longer than would otherwise be the case to keep the organs "fresh" for transplant.[30] May physicians keep a patient in a "vegetable" state indefinitely, awaiting use for his organs?

The only helpful scriptural guideline I know for such cases is the Golden Rule: Do unto others as you would have them do unto you (Matt. 7:12). Certainly, a patient has the right to stipulate that in the event of his imminent death, his body may be preserved indefinitely as needed for transplant purposes. That could be a "praiseworthy" act in terms of our earlier analysis. But may the physician impose this situation upon a patient *without* his informed consent? If I were a physician, I would not feel free to do so. The idea of living indefinitely as a "vegetable" is repugnant to me, and, I suspect, to most of us. I would not wish to impose that kind of existence upon anyone without his consent. I would see that sort of existence as a major sacrifice on the part of the patient (and his family!),

29. Here I am indebted to Greg Bahnsen's lectures on medical ethics, which are available on tape from Geneva Ministries, Box 131300, Tyler, TX 75713. Bahnsen's lectures discuss these passages in more detail.

30. Of course there is also an opposite problem with transplant technology, namely the danger of removing someone from life-support *too soon* to make his organs available to someone else. See section B above, end.

one that the patient has a right to make but that no one else may make for him.

If we are not talking about "indefinite" preservation, however, but about preserving the patient for a relatively short period of time (maybe a week or two), then I would not have the same problem. Again, the Golden Rule is the operative principle. Speaking for myself, I would not like to be kept in a vegetable state for a year, awaiting transplant usage; I certainly would not object to being kept in that state for a couple of weeks, if that would result in bringing help to someone in serious need. This is a vague guideline of course. The Golden Rule is a very "existential" principle, one that varies in its application from person to person. Someone else may apply it very differently than I, and care providers must follow their own consciences, not mine. What I have said does, however, illustrate the *type* of thinking that must be done in the situation.

D. LIVING WILLS

A living will is a legal document wherein someone stipulates that extraordinary means not be used to keep him alive should hope of recovery be gone and he is incompetent to make his wishes known.[31] Such documents are intended to avoid unduly prolonging the dying process, with its attendant enormous expense and emotional frustration. That desire, in biblical terms, is legitimate, even commendable. As we have said, one should be allowed to die once dying actually begins, and even before that point, one might legitimately sacrifice himself by refusing maximal efforts to prolong his life.

There are, however, questions as to whether the living will is a good instrument for this purpose.

a. The distinction between ordinary and extraordinary care, as we have indicated, is not precise. What is "extraordinary" depends on the particular situation or injury or disease. But that is precisely what is unknown at the time the living will is signed. Differences of religious or philosophical perspective between physician and

31. Cf. John Jefferson Davis, *Evangelical Ethics* (Phillipsburg, N.J.: Presbyterian and Reformed Publishing Co., 1985), 184.

patient may lead the physician to interpret the living will in a way not intended by the patient.

b. "Hope of recovery" is also imprecise. Does it mean restoration of consciousness or of a certain "quality of life"? Of course an actual legal document may try to be more precise; but attempts at greater precision often create, paradoxically, even more problems of interpretation. And if we make the document *too* precise, we may remove from the physician exactly the flexibility he needs to respond adequately in a crisis.

c. A person's intentions when writing a living will may be different from what his desires turn out to be in an actual crisis. A physician, therefore, can have no assurance that in carrying out the provisions of the living will he is carrying out what the patient, if conscious, would actually desire. Bahnsen, in his previously mentioned lectures on medical ethics, poses the following question: What if the patient were to wake up in the hospital and say, "Wait, don't let me die!"? Since it is always possible that a patient will change his mind, how can a physician be sure that he is doing what the patient would want done if the patient were conscious and competent to make decisions concerning his welfare? But the whole purpose of the living will is to provide the physician with a knowledge of the patient's true intent and wishes.

d. The living will, vague as its language often is, may create legal snarls, demands for court rulings, fears of malpractice litigation, and similar problems that may inhibit the exercise of medical judgment and the speedy administration of proper care. Of course, such snarls arise without living wills, though living wills are intended to avoid such problems. For those reasons, living wills may not be good instruments.

Davis notes that the "durable power of attorney," which is recognized in forty-one states, is an alternative to the living will.

> [The durable power of attorney] allows a person to designate an individual who would act on his behalf should he become physically or mentally unable to make such decisions. Such an arrangement meets the fears of "overtreatment," without reducing the physician's flexibility to provide the optimal medical care given the specifics of a particular terminal illness.[32]

32. Ibid., 185.

The purpose of the durable power of attorney is to give legal authority to a designated proxy in addition to moral authority that the proxy has by virtue of family, church, or other ties. The legal sanction gives the proxy somewhat more power in the situation: physicians will more readily accept the desires of one who has formal legal authority than of one who does not.

The durable power of attorney also has advantages over the living will. A living person is more flexible, more responsive to circumstances, than is a paper document. He can interpret his own words, while a document must be interpreted by others. The "attorney," however, faces one of the same problems we have seen in the document: he is not an infallible guide to the *present* wishes of the patient.

His *power*, therefore, should not be greater than that of any other proxy. He should not assume the right to impose on a patient some self-sacrificial act to which the patient himself had not consented.[33]

CONCLUSION

We have seen, I trust, some of the complications of ethical decision making and some of the special resources available to Bible-believing Christians for resolving difficult ethical questions. But an evangelical commitment to Scripture does not entail that all difficult ethical problems have "easy answers." On the contrary, we have seen that sometimes Evangelicals must work even harder than non-Evangelicals in analyzing ethical issues because Evangelicals must strive to see *precisely* how *Scripture* bears on particular moral questions. If Evangelicals could contentedly appeal to a vague standard of "justice" or "love," their process of ethical decision making would often be easier! And, of course, it is not only the case that ethical theory is difficult to formulate. Often the hardest thing is *doing* what we believe to be right, for apart from God's grace, we do not *want* to do God's will.

33. See the earlier discussion of that point.

Evangelical ethics, then, can be difficult in theory and in practice. But it is comforting and helpful to know that we do have an objective standard in Scripture and that it gives us clear guidance whenever the decision concerns our responsibility before God. And Scripture answers our practical needs as well. For it tells us of Jesus, who died that our sins might be forgiven and who rose from the dead to give us, through the Holy Spirit, the power to do right (Rom. 8:4)—but that is the subject of another book. For now, let us be thankful that God, the sovereign Lord, has given us a word concerning Himself that coheres perfectly with the situations we find in the world He created. And let us ask Him for wisdom (James 1:5) that we may come to see that coherence more perfectly.

APPENDIX A

RECENT CRITIQUES OF THE BRAIN-DEATH CRITERION

My book contains a highly qualified endorsement of the use of the cessation of brain-function as one criterion (among others) of the occurrence of death. I intended my discussion of this topic to be conservative. My main concern is to guard against the possibility of living patients being declared dead for ulterior purposes—for example, so that their organs may be "harvested" for transplanting. Nevertheless, my position may not be sufficiently conservative for some recent writers who oppose all reference to brain-function in defining what is meant by "death." Since those writers explicitly base their positions on Judeo-Christian values, we should take their concerns seriously. Some articles that propound this viewpoint have been collected in a booklet "On Understanding Brain Death," which was edited by Paul A. Byrne, M.D., and Paul M. Quay, S.J., Ph.D.[1] Their arguments may be summarized in the following points.

1. Omaha: Nebraska Coalition for Life Educational Trust Fund, n.d., but it refers to events and publications as recent as 1983.

1. Loss of brain function does not necessarily involve the destruction of the brain. The latter, of course, generally follows the former, but

> ... Safar et al. have recently begun successful brain resuscitation in cases where both brain-related criteria and the older, generally accepted ones would have justified a declaration of death. Once again, it is the existence of the organ that is primarily significant, not its functioning.[2]

2. Therefore,

> A cessation of function without altered structure does not indicate anything regarding the return of function. Hence in a determination of death there must be evidence of destruction, over and above cessation of function.[3]

Just as loss of brain function does not necessarily indicate destruction of the brain, so it does not indicate that the patient has died. Loss of brain function may lead to death, but it is not a criterion of death.

Here the authors offer some analysis of a conceptual sort: What do we mean by "brain-function"? There is, they point out, no single function that goes by that name; the brain has many functions. This is important because, in their view, advocating a brain-death criterion presupposes that the brain is the "organ of the whole," an organ with the single function of giving life to the organism. Byrne and the other writers dispute this point on scientific grounds and find it to be based on a materialistic and/or pragmatic philosophy.[4]

3. Empirically, too, they find the brain-death criterion wanting. People who are "brain dead" may have heartbeat, respiration, normal color, normal body temperature, perspiration, kidney function, and reflexes. A female patient, though "brain dead," may continue to nurture a child in her womb. All of these are different from the condition that we regard empirically as death.[5]

2. Byrne and Quay, 12.
3. Ibid., 25.
4. Ibid., 9-11.
5. Ibid., 33.

"Brain-dead" patients do sometimes recover. Are we to assume that such recoveries are resurrections from the dead?[6]

4. The UDDA[7] formulation of the brain-death criterion refers to "irreversible" cessation of brain function. But, argue Byrne and the other writers, irreversibility is a "nonempirical condition."[8] One cannot observe it, and therefore it cannot function in a criterion of death. Of course, one would have a strong case for irreversibility if the organ were actually destroyed. "But it is the manifest destruction of the brain that convinces us of this total irreversibility, not vice versa." Short of such destruction, conditions that are presently irreversible may well in the future become reversible. In the past, overdoses of certain drugs that caused cessation of brain activity were irreversible. Today, however, doctors and scientists have found ways to reverse these conditions. Quay says, "There is serious doubt about the possibility of a sound diagnosis that the brain has irreversibly ceased to function."[9] Often the presence of drugs can lead to such a diagnosis when in fact the patient can recover, and, "It is often impossible to find out whether such drugs or other conditions are present or absent."[10]

5. Against the UDDA, the authors make the point that

the booklet published by the President's Commission defines the "functions of the entire brain" as those that are relevant to the diagnosis [and] are those that are clinically ascertainable. Thus, any kind of stringency that was intended has been reduced to "relevant" and "clinically ascertainable."[11]

6. Several times these authors make it clear that they are not advocating that "everyone must have respiration supported by a ventilator before death" nor "that a ventilator cannot be removed until there is putrefaction or gangrene." Furthermore, they "are not opposed to organ transplantation."[12]

6. Cf. Ibid., 9.
7. Uniform Determination of Death Act, 1983.
8. Byrne and Quay, 13.
9. Ibid., 35.
10. Ibid.
11. Ibid., 30.
12. Ibid.

7. Instead of the brain-death criterion of the UDDA, Byrne suggests that the following formulation be enacted as law:

> No one shall be declared dead unless the circulatory and respiratory systems and the entire brain have been destroyed. Such destruction shall be determined in accord with universally accepted medical standards.[13]

I have much sympathy for the Byrne-Quay position. These men are trying to maintain Christian values against materialism and pragmatism. They are (here as in their position against abortion) trying to influence their readers to take human life more seriously. And they emphasize in their articles the importance of making sharper distinctions between coma, dying, and death, distinctions that are, of course, important concerns in this book.

Still, in my view their approach raises too many unanswered questions for their position to be fully cogent. First, though their position rests heavily on the concept of the "destruction" of the brain, nowhere in their volume do they define this concept. Einstein's brain, I understand, has been studied for many years in a somewhat preserved state. According to the Byrne-Quay view, is Einstein's brain "intact"? Byrne and the other writers say that

> destruction of a human organism does not require that the individual be changed to dust, water, or the basic chemicals of which the body is composed. However, it is not adequate to accept death in the context of absent function, even if the absent function is said to have irreversibly ceased.[14]

Those words tell us what destruction is not, but they do not define what it is. Recall their earlier statement that they do not advocate maintaining respiration until putrefaction sets in. Does that mean that a patient can be dead before he becomes gangrenous or putrefactous? The authors don't say one way or another, but they should.

Normally, when we speak of the "destruction" of an organ—when we are not thinking of its being changed to dust or being squashed

13. Ibid., 28.
14. Ibid., 42.

to bits or decaying or something similar—we determine destruction by absence of function. A heart is destroyed if it no longer pumps blood, though it may still look like a good heart. We say that a camera is broken if it no longer takes pictures, even if we personally cannot *see* anything wrong with it. Lenin, I am told, appears quite intact in his Soviet mausoleum.[15] Up to a point Byrne admits the cogency of this sort of argumentation. He says, "Documentation of the destruction of the systems can be based on absent function but only as it relates to destruction."[16] So loss of function does, after all, play a role in our judgment that the patient has died, "But only as it relates to destruction." But what does "as it relates to destruction" mean? And that, of course, is the major question. How *does* loss of function relate to destruction? To clarify that relation, we need to know what destruction is and how it differs from mere loss of function, but we don't learn that from Byrne and the other writers.

I suspect that these writers are not quite as empiricist as they try to appear. I suspect that behind their argument lies some Thomistic-Aristotelian substance philosophy. If so, that philosophical tradition might have led them to reason in this manner: The person is not dead, regardless of his inactivity, until his *substance*—what he really is, what underlies all his functions—is gone. In Thomism, activities and functions are "accidents"—nonessential and peripheral to a person's real being. A person's *substance* is something altogether different from activities and functions. But substance philosophy always runs into trouble when it tries to define what that underlying substance is. And I find the same problem in Byrne and Quay.

Byrne and Quay's arguments about irreversibility correctly portray it as a nonempirical condition that often is difficult to determine. Nevertheless, we can hardly escape having to make some judgment about it. I have no doubt that some people were declared dead in biblical times who could have been resuscitated had they lived in the era of modern medicine. Scripture does not portray

15. One of my correspondents tells me that Lenin is mostly plastic these days. But I'm sure I wouldn't know it to look at him.
16. Byrne and Quay, 42.

that as a tragedy but instead warrants regarding people as dead when their vital signs have ceased and it seems impossible to restore them on the basis of presently available knowledge and technology. I don't think we can postpone burial indefinitely on the ground that perhaps some future technology will arise that will restore the patient in question. Perhaps in the future we will find that even rigor mortis is reversible! But I don't believe that we have to anticipate the future direction of medicine to conscientiously recognize death. Sometimes, however, Byrne and Quay seem to be saying that we must.

In my view, the authors' strongest point is the empirical comparison between what is called "brain-death" and what we all recognize as death (3, above). But the problem is this: obviously the empirical signs of death (cessation of circulation and respiration, etc.) can be postponed, sometimes indefinitely, by artificial means. But does a patient ever reach a point where he is *merely* a machine that is being manipulated by other machines and is not really alive? I wish the authors had addressed this issue. I believe their position would have provided a cogent answer, something like this: If we suspect such a condition, we may remove the life support devices; but the patient should not be declared dead until he actually manifests the empirical signs of death.

In the final analysis, my position is really not different from theirs. I prefer to express the point about the relation of the condition of the brain to death without using the categories of substance philosophy. And I am not averse to defining "destruction" in terms of the irreversible loss of certain functions. What functions? In my definition of death, I include functions such as respiration, circulation, brain activity, plus such less central (but, in this case, confirming-the-hypothesis) functions as body temperature, color, kidney function, and so forth. So in practice my position works out in approximately the same way that theirs does.

As indicated in the text of this book, I am more friendly than the authors are to the *verbal formulation* of the UDDA. Earlier, however, I did criticize the UDDA for giving us the choice between two different syndromes as bases for declarations of death. I think that if circulation or respiration or brain activity (all of it!) has ceased and if that cessation is truly irreversible, then that would indicate that the "destruction" that Byrne and Quay have in mind has indeed taken place. Their point 5 (concerning the explanatory booklet), however, keeps me from wholeheartedly endorsing the UDDA. Apparently, the UDDA doesn't *really* mean that *all* brain activity must cease. Rather, it means that only that brain activity that is traditionally observed in medical practice must have ceased. Or should we consider the UDDA booklet to be less authoritative than the actual text of the UDDA? The confusion, in any case, weakens the value of the UDDA as model legislation or practical guideline.

Thus I am in general agreement with Byrne and Quay, though our rhetoric is different and I find them guilty of some confusion—or at least they have been unable completely to remove my own confusion about their position.

APPENDIX B

REPORT OF THE COMMITTEE TO STUDY THE MATTER OF ABORTION[1]

1988 PREFACE TO THE COMMITTEE'S REPORT ON ABORTION

In 1970 I was appointed to a committee that the General Assembly of the Orthodox Presbyterian Church created to study the matter of abortion. I was the principal author of the committee's *Report* (though I received valuable help from the other committee members), which was approved by the assembly of 1972, the 1971 assembly having postponed consideration. It was rather unusual for a General Assembly of the O.P.C. to "approve" or "adopt" any statement on social ethics. A substantial minority of delegates disapproved of any such statements on principle, and many of the delegates protested the vote of 1972. That the O.P.C. General Assembly nevertheless approved the *Report* shows their deep con-

1. Presented to the Thirty-eighth General Assembly of the Orthodox Presbyterian Church, May 24-29, 1971.

cern over this particularly important problem, a concern that over-
rode the Assembly's traditional stance toward social issues.

In the historic Roe versus Wade case of 1973, the Supreme Court
legalized abortion in all fifty states. That decision came as a great
shock to the evangelical world, which until then had not realized
how radically the secularist spirit had penetrated the American legal
system. Roe versus Wade became a potent symbol of the secularist
spirit and a symbol that mobilized Evangelicals into a united effort
seldom seen in our denominationally fragmented age. A strong
anti-abortion consensus, which had not existed at all in the fifties
and sixties, developed among Evangelicals and gave rise to a steady
stream of literature on the subject, a stream that still continues.

Although the O.P.C. *Report* antedates the Roe versus Wade decision (and so is outdated in some ways), and though Evangelicals
have written a great deal about abortion in the last fifteen years, I
believe that the *Report* is valuable and worthy of inclusion in this
book because it still contains one of the most elaborate *exegetical*
treatments of abortion.[2] And to Evangelicals, exegesis is always
the bottom line.[3] I hope that the *Report* continues to prove valuable to those who seek God's answer to the question of abortion.

Although I would like to rewrite the *Report* to bring some of its
sections up to date, that is not possible. The *Report* is not mine; it
is the work of a committee and ultimately is the property of the
O.P.C. It is theirs to revise if they choose. Nevertheless, I should
preface the text with some comments that indicate how I *would*
revise the *Report* were I to do so today.

For one thing, I would probably adopt a slightly more popular
style! As I reread the report, I am amazed at how much my style
was influenced in those days by the latinated prose of my late and
beloved teacher, John Murray.

Questions of style notwithstanding, however, I would change
nothing in the first twelve sections of the *Report*. The discussion of

2. I trust that readers will forgive the pride I feel when I remember that on the
topic of abortion, my denomination provided pioneering leadership to other
Evangelicals (I wish that the O.P.C. took such a role more often!).

3. The exegetical discussion in the *Report* continues to influence the writing of
other Evangelicals on the subject. Compare the *Report* with the discussions of
John Jefferson Davis in his valuable book *Abortion and the Christian* (Phillipsburg,
N.J.: Presbyterian and Reformed Publishing Co., 1984). See especially pp. 35-62.

Exodus 21:22-25 in section 13 deserves some rethinking, but perhaps I would not actually change that either. I have been greatly impressed by Meredith G. Kline's "Lex Talionis and the Human Fetus,"[4] which interacts with extrabiblical ancient Near Eastern languages and literature in a way that is beyond my competence. Kline argues that both in Case A (v. 22) and in Case B (vv. 23-25) the crime is subject to the death penalty and that therefore destruction of either mother or unborn child is a capital crime. The argument manifests Kline's usual creativity and rigor, but I do not find it entirely persuasive. The exegesis of the Report still seems to me to render the Hebrew text in the most natural way. Of course, Kline's exegesis, like that of the Report, comes to a strongly pro-life conclusion; so one who prefers Kline's treatment will not differ from the conclusions of the Report.

I would like to rewrite the language of 13, o, which addresses the present normativity of Old Testament law. Although I eschew the partisanship and jargon of the "Christian Reconstruction Movement," and though I find their argumentation sometimes (but usually not!) simplistic, I have learned from them the fundamental principle that all of God's Word is normative for us today (Matt. 4:4; 5:17-20). There are, of course, genuine questions about how the specific applications of Scripture change from age to age. I do not offer animal sacrifices or abstain from pork, nor do most of the Christian Reconstructionists.[5] But in the case of Exodus 21:22-25, I see no reason to deny the present normativity of its teaching. It seems to me quite simply to indicate God's valuation on the life of a pregnant woman and her child, a valuation that remains the same in all times and places.

In section 14, the Report mentioned twenty-eight weeks as the commonly accepted point of "viability." Since 1970, however, fetuses have lived outside of the womb twenty-two weeks after conception. Also, babies have been conceived outside the womb and

4. Journal of the Evangelical Theological Society 20, 3 (1977): 193-201.
5. For expositions of Christian Reconstructionism, see R. J. Rushdoony, The Institutes of Biblical Law (Phillipsburg, N.J.: Presbyterian and Reformed Publishing Co., 1973), reviewed by me in the Westminster Theological Journal 38:2 (Winter, 1976): 195-217; Greg Bahnsen, Theonomy in Christian Ethics (Phillipsburg, N.J.: Presbyterian and Reformed Publishing Co., 1977, 1984).

later implanted therein. It is more and more evident that future technology will make it possible to raise children from conception entirely outside of the womb. When that happens, the point of "viability" will be zero weeks.

Sections 15 and 16 deserve some rethinking too. Kenneth Gentry, particularly, has suggested that an argument could be developed that is less dependent on burden of proof and probability considerations. I am not entirely convinced that can be done, but if it could be, that would doubtless be an advantage. Still, I continue to maintain the fundamental point: even if you have some doubt that the unborn child is a person, you are biblically obligated to give to the child the *benefit* of the doubt. Since many will continue to be in doubt no matter how cogent our arguments, that point deserves continual emphasis.

Section 17 contains many statistics that are, of course, very much outdated. The present situation, in which abortion is always legal, is very different from the situation in 1970, in which anti-abortion laws were common. Still, I know of no recent statistics that call into question the conclusions of section 17, and most of the recent statistics that I have seen reinforce those conclusions significantly.

Section 18, *a* argues that in some cases it is legitimate for governments to restrict religious freedoms. I would now put the point more strongly: all law, when legitimate, restricts freedom of religion! Why? Because all crime is the expression of religious rebellion against God and against His social institutions (such as government). Thus criminal behavior is a form of practical unbelief and so is functionally equivalent to adopting a false theology. Civil law, when it is working properly, *always* restricts the exercise of that sort of practical unbelief, of that sort of false religion. Therefore Christians should not be embarrassed when their opposition to abortion is described as "religious." It is, of course, precisely that. Therefore attempts to portray or categorize the issue of abortion as "moral, not religious" or as "scientific, not religious" weaken the central thrust of our Christian concern about abortion. (Incidentally, we can see from the preceding argument how silly and illogical it is to assert some absolute separation between religious and civil matters.)

PREFACE

Each day it becomes more and more urgent for the church to speak a word from God concerning the current drive for liberalized abortion laws. If abortion is sin in any sense, then we should be most concerned about the breadth and depth of the desire for it in our culture. And if abortion is murder, even in some cases, then the current pace of abortion liberalization could lead to a slaughter of defenseless human beings worse than the atrocities of Hitler, Stalin, or Herod the Great.

Yet Christians have been reluctant to address this issue boldly and forthrightly. Apart from the carnal timidity that inhibits Christian witnessing on *all* issues, this reluctance may be ascribed largely to two difficulties: (1) the difficulty of demonstrating from Scripture that the unborn child is, from conception, a human person whose right to life is protected by the sixth commandment and (2) the difficulty of reconciling the rights of the unborn (however they be construed) with other concerns for which we find scriptural basis. Thus Christians have been tempted to back away from the abortion controversy, perhaps even to rest in the false consolation that our present ignorance concerning the matter will excuse us of blame for any evil resulting from our inaction. But God does not excuse slothful and willful ignorance, nor does He excuse us of complicity in evil resulting from such ignorance. He calls us in this, as in all matters, to search out the whole counsel of God, to resolve our difficulties as much as Scripture allows, and to proclaim the truth with confidence. We pray that God will use this report to help Christians resolve their problems in this area and hence to purify and embolden their testimony.

John M. Frame
Robert L. Malarkey
Joseph Memmelaar

*   *   *   *   *

In this report, *abortion* will be used to refer to any intentional killing of a human embryo or fetus. For the sake of simplicity, and to put the ethical issue at stake into sharper focus, this definition assigns to the term a broad meaning (instead of the narrower usage wherein abortion is distinguished from miscarriage and premature labor as an *early* termination of pregnancy). Further, the term will not be used to denote spontaneous abortion unless the adjective *spontaneous* accompanies it.

Concerning the "matter of abortion," then, Scripture compels us to make the following affirmations.

1. The greatest of the commandments is the law of love (Matt. 22:36-40 and parallels; John 13:34f.; Rom. 13:8-10; Gal. 5:14). Our first obligation, therefore, in any ethical decision is to manifest genuine love for God and for other people. In this context we must ask: Can a decision in favor of abortion (in general or in a particular situation) ever be an act of love? The question is a searching one; it forces us not only to dig deeply into Scripture but also to analyze the profoundest motives of our own hearts. Sometimes, however, decisions in favor of abortion are all too clear in their motivation. Sometimes the spirit of selfishness, of greed, of destruction, of hate is plain enough to be seen by all, except perhaps the one in whom that spirit dwells. When one decides in favor of abortion merely for convenience, or when a woman has an abortion simply to show that she can "do anything she wishes with her own body"—surely she is far from the spirit of the Lord Jesus Christ who humbled Himself and even laid down His life for His friends. Here the motive is obvious to anyone with a basic understanding of Scripture. To such as these we need say no more before demanding repentance.

2. Yet sometimes the motives are not so obvious. Often, motives are mixed, and the dominant motive is hard to find. Such difficulties should direct us back to the law of God for more clarification; for it is the law that shows us what love does and what loves does not do. Here, of course, we must beware of using exegesis as a means of rationalization: it is always tempting to read the law in a Pharisaic way, using it to justify our wicked hearts by pointing to the formal correctness of our actions. Yet to the Christian the law

is indispensable; it is his final authority, the very Word of God Himself. Without the law we would have no knowledge of love whatever, for love is itself a command and is defined in the context of all God's commands.

3. What, then, is the unborn child, according to Scripture? He is, first of all, a *creature of God*. Does that point seem too obvious to mention? Yet this affirmation alone is a decisive rebuke to the spirit of human autonomy. Yet the unborn child belongs (in the most ultimate sense) not to his parents, nor to human society in general, nor to government, but to God. No created thing is man's simply to use as he pleases, disregarding God's will. Man has dominion over the earth, to be sure; but this dominion was intended to be a covenant stewardship under God, not a usurpation of God's authority. Our present environmental crisis shows vividly how sin corrupts man's rightful dominion into a lustful and destructive tyranny. To say that the unborn child is ours to treat as we please is to give less consideration to the child than God demands we give to rivers and rocks.

4. But the unborn child is more than a river or a rock, more than other creatures of God: he is a *living* creature, one possessing a divinely granted sovereignty over the inanimate creation (Gen. 1). Along with other living creatures, he stands under the protection of God's covenant with Noah (Gen. 9:9f.). The blood of even subhuman living creatures had a special preciousness in the Old Testament period. Since the blood of an animal represented its divinely created *life*, such blood was not to be consumed by man (Lev. 17:14), and the shedding of it was the God-appointed means of prefiguring the atoning work of Christ (Lev. 17:11). In these ordinances, God required of His people a careful regard for the lives of all of His creatures, even those whose lives were to be sacrificed to meet the needs of man. Man's dominion over *living* creatures is even more explicitly limited in Scripture than is his dominion over the inanimate world.

5. But the unborn child is more even than a merely "living" creature: he is *human* life, and therefore a bearer of the image of God. Some indeed may wish to argue that he is not an *independent* human life because he functions as a part of his mother's body—

this argument we shall discuss later. But even if the child is not an independent human life, there can be no doubt that he is *human*— just as human, at least, as his mother's arms or legs. It must not be supposed that at some point between conception and birth the child develops uniquely human characteristics in the place of uniquely subhuman ones. From the point of conception, he has a full complement of human chromosomes and is in that respect different from every subhuman embryo or fetus. From the very beginning, he is a *human* child, and his humanity is verifiable in every cell of his body.

Now even if the unborn child were merely a part of his mother's body, he would still be a bearer of the image of God. The image of God pertains to all aspects of man's being, the physical included. According to Scripture, it is man himself, not merely some aspect of man, that is made in the image of God. This fact places the unborn child under a specific scriptural protection, for the biblical prohibition of murder is based upon the presence of the image of God in man (Gen. 9:6). And according to the Westminster Shorter Catechism, the prohibition of murder forbids not only "the taking away of our own life or the life of our neighbor unjustly" but also "whatsoever tendeth thereunto" (Q. 69), which according to the Larger Catechism includes "striking" and "wounding" (Q. 136). Since man is made in the image of God, therefore, he has no unlimited sovereignty over his own body (cf. 1 Cor. 6:15-7:4). He may not harm or wound it without just cause. To say, then, that the unborn child is part of his mother's body is not to offer an excuse for destroying him but rather to establish a presumption in favor of preserving him.

6. But still more must be said. The unborn child is not merely human life, significant though that fact may be. He is a product of the *human reproductive system*. Throughout Scripture, man's sexual life is a matter of particular divine concern. The Bible is nowhere more emphatic in its condemnation of pretended human autonomy than in its teaching concerning sex. The sacredness of the sexual relation is indicated often in Scripture: immediately following the statement that man was created in God's image, we learn of his sexual differentiation (Gen. 1:27). The first effect of sin noted in

the account of the Fall is sexual shame (Gen. 3:7, 10). The Mosaic Law not only demanded marital fidelity, it also placed ceremonial sanctions upon various sexual functions: male emissions and female menstruation, as well as the event of childbirth itself, were causes for ceremonial uncleanness (Lev. 12; 15; 18:6-23; 20:10-21). The New Testament, too, demands that sexual activity be kept within certain bounds. Its condemnation of "sins against the body" and its teaching that neither husband nor wife has "power over his own body" both occur in a context dealing specifically with sexual conduct (1 Cor. 6:15-7:7). The importance of this sexual purity is underscored by the fact that the marriage relation mirrors the relation between Christ and the church. If God is so jealous to maintain His lordship in this area of human life, is it conceivable that the product of sexual intercourse—the unborn child—should be wholly consigned to the whims of his parents?

7. Our rhetorical question must indeed be answered in the negative, for God is concerned not only with human sexual activity as such, but also with the *result* of that activity in the *conception of children*. Man's reproductive function plays a crucial role both in man's cultural task (Gen. 1:28, the command to be fruitful and multiply) and in the promise of redemption (which is from the outset of redemptive history the promise of *seed*, Gen. 3:15). The faith of Eve is demonstrated particularly in connection with her childbearing (Gen. 4:1, 25). The Abrahamic (Gen. 15:1-5) and the Davidic (2 Sam. 7:12-16) covenants contain explicit promises of seed, and the other Old Testament covenants presuppose such promises. The Old Testament abounds in genealogies, demonstrating the historical development of the "seed of the promise" through the birth of children, a development that reaches its culmination in the birth of Christ (Matt. 1:1-17; Luke 3:23-38). It is in this context that we should understand the biblical regulation of sexual activity (above, section 6) and also the profound conviction of the biblical saints that conception was a precious gift of God while barrenness was a curse (Gen. 4:1, 25; 21:1f.; 25:21; 29:31-35; 30:17-24; 33:5; Deut. 7:13; 28:4; Judg. 13:2-7; 1 Sam. 1:1-20; Ruth 4:13; Pss. 113:9; 127:3-5; 128:1-6; Isa. 54:1; Luke 1:24, in a more profound sense, cf. Matt. 1:20; Luke 1:31). Although the physical gene-

alogy of the redemptive line ends in Christ, the New Testament continues to regard the children of believers as a spiritual as well as a temporal blessing. God still carries out His redemptive purposes through the drawing of households to Himself (Acts 11:14; 16:15; 16:31-34; 18:8), the children of which are "holy" (1 Cor. 7:14). God has, therefore, a definite, personal, even redemptive concern with the event of conception, for by conception He has determined to bless His people and to build up His kingdom on earth. In this context the question of abortion becomes: In what cases, if ever, is it legitimate for us to destroy what God has created to bless His people and to build up His church? Also: In what cases, if ever, is the attitude of one planning abortion compatible with the biblical "joy in conception"? These questions are not entirely rhetorical; we have not yet answered them as fully as they can be answered. Yet, asked in the right spirit, they provide an important context for our thinking on this issue.

8. But God is not only active in the event of conception itself. He is directly involved in all aspects of the child's development *between conception and birth*. In Psalm 139:13-16 David reflects on the amazing knowledge and wisdom by which God formed his body in the womb of his mother. (Note that v. 16 contains the only occurrence in Scripture of the Hebrew term *golem*, embryo or fetus.) In Jeremiah 1:5 the prophet is said to be "formed in the belly" of his mother by God. (In this connection see Job 31:15; Ps. 119:73; Eccl. 11:5.) The gestation period is ruled throughout by God's providence and care. To those considering abortion, therefore, we must ask: When, if at all, does man have the right to interrupt this marvelous exhibition of God's wisdom and concern?

9. Still further: prenatal death is in Scripture regarded as a particularly terrible form of the *curse* that rests upon man because of sin. God threatens Israel with precisely this curse because of their faithlessness (Hos. 9:14) and conversely promises to bless His people (not only with conceptions, but) with live births as a consequence of obedience (Exod. 23:26). Upon the wicked, God's judgment is that they shall be "as an untimely birth" (Ps. 58:8). One of the worst things that can be said of a man in Scripture is that he is no better than an untimely birth (Job 3:10-16; 10:18f.; Eccl. 6:3; cf.

Matt. 26:24; Mark 14:21; Jer. 20:14-18). In 1 Corinthians 15:8, Paul
uses the term *ektroma*, "untimely birth" (perhaps as it had been used
by his critics—it occurs only here in Scripture), to acknowledge
dramatically the "unnaturalness," the "unexpectedness," the "in-
appropriateness" of his apostolic calling. Paul had not followed
Jesus through His earthly ministry, nor had he witnessed the origi-
nal Resurrection appearances, nor heard Jesus' teaching during the
"forty days," nor witnessed the Ascension. Rather, after these great
events Paul had set himself against Christ, persecuting the church.
Thus God appeared to him, not as to one prepared by his faithful
participation in this redemptive history to preach the gospel, but
as to one spiritually dead, untimely born, "aborted." Here, as
throughout Scripture, death before birth is an object of horror, a
result of curse, a consequence of sin. In this context the abortion
question becomes: When, if at all, does man have the right, not
only to interrupt God's prenatal care for the unborn, but to interrupt this process in order to impose upon the child that fate that is
almost a paradigmatic emblem of divine curse?

10. Yet more: Scripture assumes a *significant personal continuity
between prenatal and postnatal human life*. In Psalm 139:13 David
sees *himself* as existing in his mother's womb: "For thou didst form
my inward parts: Thou didst cover *me* in my mother's womb." In
Jeremiah 1:5 similar language is used, this time with God Himself
as the speaker: "Before I formed *thee* in the belly I knew *thee*, and
before *thou* camest out of the womb I sanctified *thee* . . ." (emphasis
ours here and in all scriptural citations). It was Jeremiah himself in
the womb that God was forming, and God was forming him with a
view toward the carrying out of his adult responsibilities. In the
New Testament we learn that John the Baptist, while still in his
mother's womb (in the sixth month of her pregnancy or later—cf.
Luke 1:24, 26) responded to the salutation of Mary in a way befit-
ting the character of his later ministry (Luke 1:41, 44). This event
should not, of course, be construed as the natural, usual course of
events; clearly the incident is an extraordinary sign of Jesus' lordship. Yet it presupposes the sort of continuity between prenatal life
that we have noted above: John in the womb is called *brephos*, a
babe, and is said to have leaped "for joy." Such is indeed the gen-

eral pattern of scriptural usage; for those in the womb are commonly referred to in Scripture by the same language used of persons already born (cf. Gen. 25:22; 38:27ff.; Job 1:21; 3:3, 11ff.; 10:18f.; 31:15; Isa. 44:2, 24; 49:5; Jer. 20:14-18; Hos. 12:3; see also the references below). At the very least, this continuity indicates that God is not only forming and caring for the unborn child; He is forming him as a specific individual, to fit him specifically for his postnatal calling. This continuity is a warning against distinguishing with careless sharpness between fetal and infant life. And the abortion question now becomes: When, if at all, has man the right to destroy an unborn child, thereby cutting off the life of an individual who is being divinely prepared to play a particular role in God's world?

11. And: that personal continuity extends back in time *to the point of conception*. Psalm 51:5 clearly and strikingly presses this continuity back to the point of conception. In this passage David is reflecting on the sin in his heart that had recently taken the form of adultery and murder. He recognizes that the sin of his heart is not itself a recent phenomenon but goes back to the point of his conception in the womb of his mother: "And in sin did my mother conceive me." The personal continuity between David's fetal life and his adult life goes back as far as conception, and extends even to this ethical relation to God!

12. Yet in order to present the matter as clearly as possible, it must also be said that there is also a personal continuity that extends from adult life backwards in time even *before conception and into eternity*. God knew Jeremiah, not only after his conception but even before it: "*Before* I formed thee in the belly I knew *thee*" (Jer. 1:5). The incarnate Son of God was given His name by the angel before His actual conception, that is, before His actual incarnation (Luke 2:21). Levi is said to have paid tithes to Melchizedek while still "in the loins of" his great-grandfather Abraham (Heb. 7:9f.). All of these assertions are true because of the sovereignty of God who works all things after the counsel of His own will (Eph. 1:11). Before anyone is actually conceived in the womb, God has planned the course of his life and his eternal destiny. Of God's elect it can be said that "He chose *us* in [Christ] *before the foundation of the world*"

(Eph. 1:4). Even *before* their conception, therefore, Scripture speaks of people in the language used of persons already born. All of us, even before we "exist," have a kind of "personal existence" as ideas in the mind of God. We shall make a negative application of this principle at a later point (section *15, a,* below). At this point, however, let us note a positive implication: human life in the womb is a certain stage in the realization of an eternal plan. Even before conception, God sees, as it were, the "finished product"—the complete man with all his gifts and characteristics, in his belief or unbelief, fitted for blessing or destruction. Conception itself, as well as the gestation process, is in every aspect oriented to the fulfillment of that plan. If indeed the child should die before birth, then that is itself a result of God's plan. But such death is closely analogous to infant death (and for that matter to all human death) —for it is the death of one whom up until that point God had cared for, preserved, and blessed; and it is the death of one who, had he not died, would have grown further toward mature humanity, toward the accomplishment of mature human goals. In this light, the abortion question becomes: What human being will dare to take the responsibility for such death upon himself?

13. There is *nothing* in Scripture that even remotely suggests that the unborn child is anything *less than a human person from the moment of conception.* The only passage that has been alleged to make such a suggestion is Exodus 21:22-25, which we will now discuss in some detail. Those who use this passage to support the thesis that the unborn child is something less than a human person interpret it as follows. They see verse 22 as describing the destruction of an unborn child and find it significant that such destruction is punished only by a fine while harm done to the mother (vv. 23-25) merits more severe penalties, including the death penalty in the event of her death. On this account the passage may be paraphrased: "And if men fight together and hurt a pregnant woman so that her child dies, yet she herself is not harmed, he shall be surely fined, according as the woman's husband shall lay upon him; and he shall pay as the judges determine. But if the woman herself is harmed, then thou shalt give life for life, eye for eye, tooth for tooth, hand for hand, foot for foot, burning for burning, wound

for wound, stripe for stripe." On this view the child is given a "lesser value" than the mother and is therefore regarded as something less than a human person.

This use of Exodus 21:22-25 raises questions in the following areas: (1) the *normativity* of this piece of Old Testament civil legislation for the New Testament church, (2) the adequacy of the *interpretation* of the passage used in this argument, (3) the legitimacy of the use of the passage so interpreted to prove the *thesis* that the unborn child is something less than a human person, and (4) the legitimacy of the use of this thesis to justify in at least some cases the *practice* of abortion. We shall take up these four questions in reverse order.

a. Even if the passage does prove the thesis in question, this fact does not prove that abortion is ever justified. Even if the unborn child is something less than a human person, this status does not justify his destruction under all, or some, or even *any* circumstances. In sections *1-12* above, we have presented considerations directed against the destruction of the unborn that do not presuppose his status as a human being in the fullest sense. To justify abortion, even if we regard the unborn child as less than a person, those considerations must be refuted, or at least they must be shown to be overridden by other principles in the case in question.

b. Also relevant to question *(4)* is the teaching of the passage under consideration (granting the adequacy of the proposed interpretation). For it must not be forgotten that on any interpretation, the passage regards the destruction of the unborn as an offense, a wrong, a sin. In the absence of any other scriptural teaching that would establish exceptions to or modifications of the condemnation issued in this passage, it is perverse indeed to attempt to justify abortion by reference to a passage that condemns precisely the sort of destruction performed by the abortionist. The fact that there is, on the proposed interpretation in question, a lighter penalty attached to the destruction of the unborn than to harm done the mother must not be overestimated in its importance. The Christian cannot justify committing sin on the ground that his sin is less heinous than other kinds of sin.

c. Again, granting the normativity of the interpretation and thesis asserted in the argument: this passage clearly deals with a case of *accidental* killing. If even such accidental killing of an unborn child is punished by a fine, we must surely assume that the *intentional* killing of an unborn child is at least as serious as (in all probability more serious than) the offense in view in verse 22. This fact makes it all the more perverse to defend abortion (on our definition, the *intentional* destruction of the unborn) on the basis of this passage. How can we defend the *intentional* destruction of the unborn on the basis of a passage that condemns even its *accidental* destruction?

d. One must object at this point that there are other scriptural considerations that would require exceptions to the general rule given in this passage. In such an event, such consideration might be combined with the "thesis" (above, question (3)) obtained from this passage to produce a justification for a particular abortion. We are not concerned to deny such a possibility now, only to make clear that this passage, taken *in itself*, does nothing to justify any practice of abortion, even if the other questions regarding this argument can be answered satisfactorily.

e. But we must now move on to question (3). Does the passage prove the thesis that the unborn child is less than a human person, granted the proposed interpretation? The argument is that since there is a lesser penalty for destruction of the child than for harm done to the mother, the child must have been regarded as "less than a human person." But this inference is not a sound one. The rationale for the various penalties assessed in the Mosaic Law is an interesting and complicated subject, one concerning which there is much room for debate. That the disparity in punishment must be due to a disparity between personhood and nonpersonhood is an interesting thesis but one that cannot be simply assumed without argument. And there are, in our view, no arguments that render necessary such a conclusion.

f. The lack of a death penalty for destruction of the unborn in verse 22 does nothing to support the thesis in question. The law of Moses did not as a rule impose a mandatory death penalty in cases of accidental killing (cf. Exod. 21:13f., 20f.). If indeed the law does impose such a penalty for the destruction of the mother's life (v. 23, "life for life"), then we have in this passage not a devaluation of the life of the child, but an extraordinary valuation upon the life of the

mother, doubtless to give her (and her unborn child!) special protection throughout her pregnancy.

g. That there is no mention in verse 22 of an "avenger of blood"
and of "cities of refuge" (after the pattern of other passages dealing
with accidental killing, Num. 35:10-34; Deut. 9:1-13; cf. Exod.
21:13f.) does not demonstrate the thesis in question. No one
doubts that the accidental killing of an unborn child is a unique
case, one that might very well have failed to arouse the blood vengeance presupposed in the "cities of refuge" passages. The question, however, is whether this uniqueness is due to the child's lack
of personhood. And that is the question that cannot be answered
by the presence or absence of the vengeance formulae.

h. But does not the very lightness of the penalty serve to establish the thesis in question? We think not. The immediately preceding passage (Exod. 21:20f.), in fact, presents a situation where a
master who kills his slave unintentionally (the lack of intent being
proved by the interval between the blow and the death) escapes
with no penalty at all! To argue from this passage that slaves are regarded by God as less than human persons would be precarious indeed! To argue from Exodus 21:22-25 that the unborn child is not a
person is even less plausible. Doubtless the unborn child, like the
slave, had a lesser status in Israelite society than other persons. It
cannot be demonstrated, however, that this lesser status was a
status of nonpersonhood. And that is the point at issue.

i. If in spite of the above considerations we choose to regard our
passage as establishing the thesis in question, then some serious
consequences must be faced. The passage makes no distinction
between embryo and fetus, none between viable and nonviable
fetuses. All unborn children are reckoned equally in its teaching. If
this passage be taken to prove that the unborn child is less than a
person, then this conclusion must be taken to hold for *all* unborn
children, even those who have been in the womb a full nine
months! Depending on the extent to which this principle is understood as a guide to the practice of abortion, this view could result
in the killing of a child ten minutes before its expected birth on the
ground that it is not "really a person." If we accept the thesis under
discussion, then we may be forced to smother our natural repug-

nance to such a practice. It is of course true that our Scripture requires us to adopt viewpoints that are repugnant to our sensibilities, when those sensibilities are not themselves sanctified. But we should not adopt a position without facing squarely such consequences; and if they cannot be reconciled with other aspects of our sensibilities, we should turn to Scripture until the problem is resolved.

j. We now turn to question (2): Does the argument in question rest upon an adequate interpretation of Exodus 21:22-25? We answer in the negative. In the first place, the term *yeled* in verse 22 never refers elsewhere to a child lacking recognizable human form or to one incapable of existing outside the womb. The possibility of such a usage here, as the interpretation in question requires, is still further reduced by the fact that if the writer had wanted to speak of an undeveloped embryo or fetus there may have been other terminology available to him. There was the term *golem* (Ps. 139:16), which *means* "embryo, fetus." But in cases of the death of an unborn child, Scripture regularly designates him not by *yeled*, not even by *golem*, but by *nefel* (Job 3:16; Ps. 58:8; Eccl. 6:3), "one untimely born." The use of *yeled* in verse 22, therefore, indicates that the child in view is not the product of a miscarriage, as the interpretation in question supposes; at least this is the most natural interpretation in the absence of decisive considerations to the contrary. (The reason for the plural form is difficult to assess on any interpretation. If, as some have suggested, it refers to the woman's capacity for bearing, then the passage becomes quite irrelevant to the matter of abortion. If, as is more likely, it is a plural of indefiniteness, allowing for the possibility of more than one child in the mother's body, then the plurality of the term would fit as easily into our interpretation as into the interpretation under criticism.)

k. Further, the verb *yatza'* in verse 22 ("go out," translated "depart" in KJV) does not in itself suggest the death of the child in question, and is ordinarily used to describe normal births (Gen. 25:26; 38:28-30; Job 3:11; 10:18; Jer. 1:5; 20:18). With the possible exception of Numbers 12:12, which almost certainly refers to a stillbirth, it never refers to a miscarriage. The Old Testament term normally used for miscarriage and spontaneous abortion, both in humans and in animals, is not *yatza'* but *shakol* (Exod. 23:26; Hos.

9:14; Gen. 31:38; Job 2:10; cf. 2 Kings 2:19, 21; Mal. 3:11). The most natural interpretation of the phrase *weyatze'u yeladheyha*, therefore, will find in it not an induced miscarriage, not the death of an unborn child, but an induced premature birth, wherein the child is born alive, but ahead of the anticipated time.

l. We should also note that the term *ason* (harm), found in both verse 22 and verse 23 is indefinite in its reference. The expression "*lah*" (to her), which would restrict the harm to the woman in distinction from the child, is missing. Thus the most natural interpretation would regard the "harm" as pertaining either to the woman or to the child. Verse 22 therefore describes a situation where neither mother nor child is "harmed"—i.e., where the mother is uninjured and the child is born alive. Verse 23 describes a situation where some harm *is* done—*either* to mother *or* child *or* both. This point confirms the interpretation we are advocating (above, *j-k*). An induced miscarriage could hardly be described as a situation where there is "no harm." Verse 22, therefore, describes, not an induced miscarriage but an induced premature birth. A further implication of this reading of *ason*: when punishments are assessed in verses 23-25, the unborn child is protected, as is his mother, by the law of retaliation. The passage does not, of course, demonstrate that the child is given the same protection as his mother under this law; but it is clear that he is protected, that harm done to him is punished by some sort of retaliation, and thus that even his accidental destruction is wrong in the sight of God. If indeed other scriptural considerations require exceptions to this principle, then perhaps abortion might in some cases by justifiable; but this passage taken in itself offers no encouragement to any proposed abortion; on the contrary, the bearing of the passage upon the question is quite otherwise.

m. The reason for the fine in verse 22 is difficult to assess, but no more difficult on our interpretation than on any other. It is true that verse 22 does ordain a fine ('*anash*) rather than vengeance (*naqam*, as in the preceding passage, v. 20). Fines are not often assessed in the Mosaic Law. The only other occurrence of '*anash* in the Pentateuch is in Deuteronomy 22:19, where a fine is assessed upon one who had "brought up an evil name upon a virgin of Israel." Could it be that premature birth was somehow considered shameful and that the fine in Exodus 21:22, in analogy with Deuteronomy 22:19, is a kind of damages for the harm done to the woman's reputation? Equally likely, the fine could be the compensation for the trouble, expense, and danger involved in premature delivery. But to understand the precise reason for it, we would doubtless have to have a more thorough understanding of Israelite culture than we now have. On the interpretation we are opposing, a fine would be compensation for the loss of an unborn child—a rather lenient penalty, it would seem, in view of the importance given to heirs and descendants in that culture (see above, section 7), and in any case a penalty with no clear analogies elsewhere in Scripture. We are not dogmatic on this matter, but we think that the evidence available tends to confirm, rather than to disconfirm, the interpretation which we have established on the basis of considerations *j-l* above.

n. To summarize the proper interpretation of this passage, we regard the following as an adequate paraphrase: "And if men fight together and hurt a pregnant woman so that her child is born prematurely, yet neither mother nor child is harmed, he shall be surely fined, according as the woman's husband shall lay upon him; and he shall pay as the judges determine. But if either mother or child is harmed, then thou shalt give life for life, eye for eye, tooth for tooth, hand for hand, foot for foot, burning for burning, wound for wound, stripe for stripe."

o. One of our four questions remains, namely the question of the normativity of this passage for our present situation. Exodus 21:22-25 is part of the civil legislation given to Israel. Principles embedded in this legislation are not necessarily normative for New Testament believers. Consider Exodus 21:20f., the immediately preceding passage. There we read that a slave can be killed by his master without penalty if the slave remains alive a day or two after the blow. This practice hardly conforms to the New Testament ethic. Like Moses' bill of divorcement (Matt. 19:7f.), some of this civil legislation involves "sufferance for hardness of heart." No doubt this civil legislation also contains principles binding upon New Testament believers, but the question of what principles are binding requires argument of a biblico-theological nature. And concerning Exodus 21:22-25, no really decisive argument of this sort has been adduced so far. We maintain that the passage, on our interpretation, conforms to the general scriptural pattern that we have already outlined (sections 1-12). If indeed unborn children are objects of God's special providential care, then it is not surprising to find in the Mosaic Law a specific, explicit protection for them, and we should assume that *no less* protection than that should be required of New Testament believers. The interpretation we oppose, indeed, also provides a certain protection for the unborn (cf. above, section 13, b-c), and in this respect it too is in keeping with the general tone of scriptural teaching on this subject. Yet to suggest, as proponents of this interpretation do, such minimal protection is the *only* protection that should be accorded the child is to argue unhistorically, to fail to understand the character of Israelite civil legislation, as in part an accommodation to the hardness of heart of the people. Thus even if the interpretation we oppose be accepted, its relevance for the determination of our present conduct must be questioned.

p. We conclude, therefore, that Exodus 21:22-25 does not suggest that the unborn child is anything less than a human person from the point of conception. Any attempt to make the passage teach such a thesis results in insuperable difficulties of exegesis, logic, and application. Since this is the only passage alleged to provide proof of such a thesis, we conclude that there is no scriptural basis for such arguments and that unless better arguments are forthcoming we cannot regard Scripture as even remotely suggesting such a view.

14. There is no purely *scientific* proof that the unborn child is anything less than a human person from the point of conception. This fact is evident from the following considerations.

a. At the outset, it must be seriously asked whether any narrowly scientific argument could possibly, even in principle, establish whether the unborn child is or is not a human person. The question of whether the unborn child is a human person is essentially the question of whether, from God's point of view, the child has the ontological status entitling him to a full human right to life. The question is religious, metaphysical, and ethical. What mere statement of scientifically verified empirical fact could answer such a question? Does genetic independence confer upon a piece of tissue the right to life? Does physical dependence of one organism upon another deprive the first organism of its right to life? These questions reveal a certain discrepancy between scientific and ethical predications such that no scientifically obtained proposition *in itself* would appear sufficient to establish ontological status and ethical rights. On the other hand, we must affirm that scientific propositions, *taken together with* the teaching of Scripture, may indeed cast light upon our questions. Scientific information is always valuable in helping the believer to understand his situation and thereby to see the relevance of Scripture to that situation. If, for example, Scripture established quickening as the point at which personal existence begins, then the scientist's skills would be needed in order to determine whether in a given case quickening had actually taken place. But a *purely* scientific argument, an argument containing only scientific premises and no scriptural premises, must be regarded as *in principle* incapable of resolving this sort of question. Thus it is impossible to prove from scientific premises alone that the unborn child is less than a human person from the point of conception. For that matter, it should also be noted that the contrary proposition is also incapable of such proof (see below, section 15).

b. To be more specific, it cannot be argued on scientific grounds that, for example, "quickening" marks the dividing line between human personhood and lack of human personhood. Quickening is the point (generally eighteen to twenty weeks after conception, with some variation) at which the mother becomes conscious of gross movements of the fetus in the womb, and has generally been regarded as a significant turning point in the development of the child. The heartbeat of the child, however, is detectable at an earlier stage of development, and the onset of quickening is continuous with such earlier "fetal motions." Quickening is not, therefore, the kind of drastic change that could plausibly be equated with the change from nonpersonhood to personhood. Further, it is difficult to see how the medical-scientific concept of "quickening" correlates with the metaphysical-religious concept of "personhood"

and the ethical concept of "right to life." Such correlations themselves are not established by scientific evidence, but rather the
result of philosophizing that the Christian must dismiss as speculative unless confirmed by Scripture. And we have shown that such
theories cannot be confirmed by Scripture (above, section 13).

c. Nor can "viability" be established as such a dividing line,
though this is the point most often seized upon by those wishing to
draw the line at some point between conception and birth. Viability is the point at which the fetus is capable of living outside the
womb and is generally thought to occur at twenty-eight weeks
after conception. This point varies, however, and that variation
makes it difficult in some cases to determine whether a fetus is
viable or not. Further, the very definition of "viable" may very
well change with the improvement of incubation technology. The
concept, therefore, does not appear to be clear enough to be work-
able as a criterion of human personhood and human right to life.
But even if the concept were perfectly clear, we would still have the
problem of showing why it is viability that determines personhood
and right to life.

d. What of birth itself as the moment at which a fetus becomes a
person? It may certainly be argued that birth is a more momentous
event in the young life than either quickening or viability. At the
moment of birth, the child ceases to be directly dependent upon
his mother's body for his own life support. At that moment he becomes independent in a sense in that he was not previously. This
fact has led to the suggestion that before birth the child should be
regarded as part of his mother's body and that only after birth
should he be regarded as a person in his own right. This suggestion, however, is not a sound one. To allege that life-support-
dependence is inconsistent with personhood is to engage in specu-
lation. For one thing it is possible for two persons (e.g., Siamese
twins) to share the same life-support systems to some extent without either of them losing his personhood, and this fact would
count against the allegation in question. Further, the dependence
of the unborn child upon his mother's body is not a metaphysical
or necessary dependence. With the advance of medical technology
it is possible to conceive of an unborn child being transplanted

from one womb to another or being raised in an incubator from shortly after conception or even being *conceived* in an artificial womb of some kind, being thus "independent" of his mother from the very beginning. To be sure, such a child could not survive without the care of *someone*, but the same is true of infants after birth. The unborn child's dependence upon his mother, therefore, is no good argument against his personhood, for it differs only in degree from the dependence of all children upon their adult guardians. Finally, the hypothesis that life-support dependence is inconsistent with personhood is essentially a philosophical supposition (like those mentioned above in *14, b-c*) with no scriptural basis.

e. Other suggestions that have been made as the dividing line between nonpersonhood and personhood include implantation of the fertilized egg in the uterus (about one week after conception) and the point at which all organ systems are initiated (about four weeks). Some have even argued that personhood begins at some time after birth, on the ground that personhood presupposes some development of cultural consciousness and interpersonal relationships. These suggestions suffer the same basic defect as the others we have considered: they fail to show how their metaphysical and ethical conclusions arrive out of their scientific premises; and they fail to do this because they fail to recognize the role that Scripture must play in this type of discussion. We therefore conclude that there is no scientific proof that the unborn child is anything less than a human person from the point of conception; and for that matter there is none to the contrary either.

15. There is *no way to demonstrate*, either from Scripture or from science or from some combination of the two, that the unborn child *is* a human person from the point of conception. In the case of attempted demonstrations from scientific premises alone, our present point is established by considerations already set forth (above, section *14, a*). Several arguments of other types have been suggested, however, and in the following paragraphs we shall have to call these attempted demonstrations into question.

a. We have noted above (section *10*) that Scripture often speaks of unborn children in the same language used to refer to those already born. The most striking examples of this usage, perhaps, are Psalm 139:13; Jeremiah 1:5; and Psalm 51:5. As we have seen, in these passages personal pronouns are used to refer to life in the womb—"me," "my," "thou," "thee." From this premise it has been argued that these passages regard the unborn children in question as human persons, and that personhood goes back to conception. Such an argument, however, reads too much into these passages. In the first place, if the fetus were not a person from conception, it is not clear that the writers would have avoided the personal pronouns. In Psalm 139:13 and in Psalm 51:5, David is reflecting on his origins. We have established (above, section 10) a "significant personal continuity" between the unborn child and his postnatal existence. Therefore, David, in considering his relation with God, traces it back to his fetal life, back even to his conception. Naturally, he uses the terms "me" and "my"; the use of "it," whether more precise or not, would be jarring, pedantic, and pointless. These pronouns are quite natural even on the supposition that the unborn child is *not* a person from conception, and thus their use does not establish the person-from-conception thesis. In the second place, we have seen (above, section 12) that according to Jeremiah 1:5 and other passages, the "personal continuity" of a man's life extends in a sense not only back to conception but even *before* conception. Personal continuity in this sense extends into eternity, into God's eternal plan. The Lord in Jeremiah 1:5 uses the pronoun "thee" of Jeremiah even *before* his conception. Now no one would argue that Jeremiah was an existing person before his conception simply because such pronouns are used of him. Rather, before his conception, when he existed in God's mind, he was *destined to become* an existent person. Thus the use of these personal pronouns does not prove that those in the womb are, while in the womb, persons. That use proves only that in God's plan those particular fetuses were (at least) *destined to become* persons.

b. Psalm 51:5, however, requires special treatment, for it is sometimes used in a different argument from the one we have just considered. We have seen (above, section 11) that this verse traces back to conception not only David's existence but even his sin. Surely, it is argued, if David was a sinner from conception, he must have been a person—for you cannot have a person's sin without a person! This is perhaps the strongest scriptural argument in favor of the person-from-conception thesis, and can be very persuasive. Yet a closer look reveals inadequacies similar to those noted above under argument *a*. David, after all, is not reflecting upon the origin of his humanity, but upon the origin of his *sin*. And all Reformed theologians have maintained (on the basis of this very verse, along with others!) that in some senses the origin of our sin antedates the origin of our existence as persons. Ultimately, sin has its mysterious origin in the eternal plan of God; proximately, our sin begins with Adam. Adam is the origin of our sin, not only in the sense that he was the first sinner in the human race but also in the sense that the guilt and penalty of his sin is imputed immediately to every human being except Jesus of Nazareth. But we are not only guilty of Adam's first sin. For Adam's sinful nature is transmitted to his descendants by "natural generation" so that each of us enters the world with a totally depraved nature. Thus "my" sin, my personal sin, the sin for which I am guilty, exists before I do (1) in the sense that God planned eternally that I would be a sinner, (2) in the sense that Adam's first sin is credited by God to my personal account, and (3) in the sense that Adam's depravity is transmitted to me through natural generation. It is not obvious, therefore, that the origin of David's sin, according to Psalm 51:5, is coincident with the origin of his human personhood. It is quite fitting for us and would have been quite fitting for David, to trace his sinfulness back beyond his individual, personal existence to those events that determined that he would in fact be a sinner. We do not of course suppose that David was sophisticated enough at this stage of redemptive history to have analyzed this situation after the manner of Romans 5. But who can doubt that David may well have had a conviction of the individual's involvement in the depravity of the race? And if indeed David saw his sin as antedating his personal existence in any sense, if such a reading of the verse is even *possible*, then the verse cannot be used to prove that David was a person from conception.

c. Exodus 21:22-25, interpreted in the way we have urged (above, 13, *j-n*), has also been used to establish the thesis that the unborn child is a person from conception. We have ourselves argued (above, *13, l*) that the passage places the unborn child under explicit, legal protection against accidental destruction. Since mother and child are under the same protection, some would argue, the child must be there regarded as a human person. We must, however, reject this inference. The passage does not specify how the law of retaliation is to be applied. Is the child to be regarded as a part of its mother, or as a person in his own right? Either way, the *lex talionis* could apply, but it would apply differently in either case. The passage simply does not specify how the unborn child is to be treated under the law and thus does not prove either that he is, or that he is not, a human person.

d. We noted earlier (above, section *10*) that in Luke 1:41, 44 John the Baptist, then still in his mother's womb, is said to have "leaped" in the womb "for joy." Some have regarded this incident as proof that the unborn child is a human person. Yet we are unable to regard this passage as proving that all unborn children are persons from conception. The fact that the child was at least six months past conception (Luke 1:24, 26) and the patently supernatural character of the event forbid us from drawing from this passage any conclusions about the personhood of unborn children in general.

e. Another argument deals with the nature of the Incarnation. The eternal Son of God became incarnate in the event of His conception by the Holy Spirit in the womb of the Virgin Mary. Surely, it is argued, He did not cease to be a person at any time during Mary's pregnancy. Therefore we have at least an analogy suggesting that personhood goes back to conception. This analogy, however, breaks down at a crucial point. The Incarnation is a unique instance of conception in the sense that the one conceived was already a person before His conception. He was not, of course, a *human* person before conception, but He was a person, and His preexistent personality continues into His incarnate state. (We should recall the Chalcedonian formula at this point: though Christ possessed two natures, He was only one person. The doctrine of the *anhypostasia* of Christ's human nature indicates that Jesus' incarnate personality is essentially that of His preincarnate state.) Since other persons do not antedate their physical existence, we do not have the same reason to suppose that they are persons from conception that we have in the case of Christ.

f. Another argument from analogy: In 1 John 3:9, the writer speaks of our spiritual "begetting" by God. (*Gennao* should be translated "beget" rather than "bear" in this verse because of the emphasis on the "seed" that remains in those begotten.) According to that verse, spiritual begetting is itself the explanation for good conduct. One who is begotten of God will not sin. Spiritual life, therefore, begins with spiritual begetting, i.e., with spiritual conception. By analogy, it therefore seems as though physical personhood begins with physical conception. This analogy between spiritual and physical conception, however, also breaks down at the most relevant point. For in the spiritual realm there is no temporal interval between conception and birth; there is no spiritual "gestation period." Thus the spiritual situation analogous to physical reproduction lacks precisely the problematic aspect that we are here concerned to analyze. The argument, therefore, does not furnish an adequate analogy to guide our thinking in this matter.

g. Finally let us consider an argument that utilizes premises from both science and Scripture: Scripture teaches that man is a psychophysical unity—that both soul and body are essential to human personhood. Science shows us that man's body begins at conception, because at conception each embryo is endowed with its own unique set of chromosomes. If man's body begins at conception, then man's soul, and hence his personhood, must begin at conception also. The weak link in this argument is the assumed correlation between "chromosomal uniqueness" and "human body." It is natural enough to want to link these two concepts and to suppose that they originate in the same event. Yet it is precisely this correlation that needs to be proved. Can there be human tissue that is chromosomally unique, that is nevertheless not a human body (and therefore not a human person)? This is the problem that the argument fails to answer. The difficulty here is, as in section *14*, above, the difficulty of correlating a scientific concept (chromosomal uniqueness) with a metaphysical-religious concept (the demonstrably human body that implies human personhood).

16. Nevertheless, the Christian is under scriptural obligation to *act on the assumption that* the unborn child is a person from conception. To clarify this statement, let us review a bit: our previous

discussion seems to leave the Christian in an intolerable situation. On the one hand, there is no proof from Scripture (section *13*) or from science (section *14*) that the unborn child is *not* a person from conception. On the other hand, the contrary thesis, that the child *is* a person from conception, also lacks demonstrative argument. There being no demonstrative proof either way, what is the Christian to do? He must make decisions concerning abortion, and in those decisions he must assume either that the unborn child is a person or that he is not. Our position is that although Scripture furnishes no demonstrative proof in this matter, it does show us clearly what our *assumptions* in such situations must be.

a. If we begin our considerations from scratch, with no arguments in front of us, we are faced with the following alternatives: either the child is (1) a part of his mother's body, deserving the same protection accorded to other parts of her body, or he is (2) a human person in his own right, deserving the same protection as other persons, or he is (3) somewhere in between, deserving less protection than a human person but more than a mere part of his mother's body. The first alternative can be dismissed rather easily on the basis of sections 6-12, above. This conclusion is confirmed by the fact that even before fertilization, the female egg is in the process of being rejected by the woman's body. If the egg is fertilized and becomes implanted in the womb, this rejection process is ordinarily suppressed for a nine month period; but this suppression is only temporary. The mother's body continues to treat the unborn child as a piece of "foreign tissue," a parasitical organism. The event of birth may be seen as the final "rejection" of this foreign tissue by the mother's body. This relation between mother and fetus does not suggest that the child should be regarded as "part of the mother's body." Furthermore, the genetic uniqueness of the fetus (section *15*, above) distinguishes the unborn child from all other tissues of his mother's body and determines that the course of his normal development will lead to eventual separation from his mother's body. Thus neither from a theological nor from a medical point of view are we entitled to regard the unborn child as a mere part of his mother's body.

b. The second alternative can neither be demonstrated nor disproved (above, sections *13-15*). Yet its *possibility* (unlike the possibility of *(1)*) cannot be discounted. The third alternative cannot be demonstrated or disproved either (above, same sections), so we are faced with a wide range of possibilities, the "somewhere" of *(3)* being indefinite and covering a number of alternatives. In a situation of this sort, the most crucial question becomes the question of *burden of proof*. Should we treat the unborn child as a human person in the absence of arguments to the contrary, or should we adopt a position in the range of *(3)* in the absence of any demonstration of *(2)*? Should we afford the unborn child maximum protection in the absence of arguments for anything less? Or may we take it upon ourselves to give him less than maximum protection on the ground that *(2) may* not be the case? When the issue is placed in such terms, we believe that the Christian will perceive an obligation to adopt *(2)* as his working assumption, that he will choose to give maximum protection to the unborn child, that he will choose in favor of life, when the issue is a matter of life and death. If there is any genuine possibility that the unborn child is, at any point, a human person made in the image of God, then the Christian cannot assume otherwise, for to do so would be to risk breaking the sixth commandment. And the risk is of a special kind. It is not as if there were some evidence tending to legitimize the killing of unborn children (on the ground of their lack of personal human status) and equal evidence tending to call such killing in question. There is nothing in Scripture that even suggests the legitimacy of such killing (cf. above, section *13*), and there is much in Scripture that calls it in question (sections *1-12, 13, 1*). Everything Scripture says on the matter has the force of *protecting* the child, and nothing in Scripture has the force of expressly limiting that protection. If indeed, as we maintain, Scripture does not say expressly *how much* protection the child deserves, must we not assume that the child should receive maximum protection until someone is able to demonstrate otherwise? Only unscriptural and arbitrary arguments have so far been offered in favor of limiting this protection below the maximum. Therefore we regard maximum protection for the unborn child as a scriptural obligation; and by "maximum" we mean treating the unborn child as a human person.

c. The same point may be made from a somewhat different perspective. Christians have always opposed infanticide on the ground of the sixth commandment. A child, say, five minutes after birth, has always been recognized by Christians as a person in the image of God, deserving of utmost care for the preservation of his life. But what of a child five minutes before birth? The child is not drastically different from the child already born, except that he happens to be still in the womb. He might, in fact, already be living outside the womb if the physician had decided to remove him surgically. The fact that he is in the womb rather than outside seems to be a small matter on which to rest a decision between life and death. Surely this child deserves the same protection, the same respect as the first child we mentioned. But what of a child ten minutes before his birth? or twenty? or five days? or three months? or six months? At what point do we abandon our high regard for the child's status in the sight of God? At what point do we decide to give him less than maximum protection? Arguments have been offered, to be sure, to the effect that this maximizing of the child's status should begin at some point in the gestation period, but such arguments are far from convincing (see above, section 14). And some argument is surely needed. An arbitrary decision in a matter of life and death is an impossibility. If someone argues for the destruction of an organism on the premise that it is not a human person, surely he must be obligated to prove that premise; he may not claim the right to assume it arbitrarily. In the absence of such argument, that is, in our present situation, the Christian has no choice but to maintain his maximal concern for the young life from conception onward. The Christian, therefore, must act on the assumption that the unborn child is a person in the sight of God and therefore under the protection of the sixth commandment.

17. Does this assumption rule out abortion under all circumstances? Not automatically. The sixth commandment as interpreted by the rest of Scripture does not forbid all killing of human beings in all situations. Scripture in fact even authorizes the destruction of human life in cases of just war and lawful capital punishment. The question is still open, therefore, as to whether there are special circumstances that would ever justify the destruction of an unborn child, granted the presumption that the child has the same right to live as other human beings. A fetus could never, of course, be subject

to capital punishment since he could never be legally convicted of a crime. In the wartime situation, the killing of unborn children must be seen in the same category as the killing of other civilians. But there are other circumstances that are sometimes claimed to make abortion necessary and that require special discussions.

a. The first argument is that abortion is necessary *as a form of population control*, if we are to avert a crisis of overpopulation. But however great the crisis may appear, and however great may be the desirability of birth control procedures, it is still not clear why this situation ever justifies abortion. There are other methods of combating overpopulation (both through birth control and through economic reorganization), and it is not clear that such methods require abortion as a supplement in order to be effective. In any case, there is no more ground for abortion as a means of population control that there is for infanticide on the same grounds.

b. Similarly, we must reject the argument that abortion is sometimes necessitated purely by the *economic* situation of the family. The Christian is indeed under obligation to consider the needs of the poor, to sympathize with and help those in economic need. But this does not mean that Christians must accept any and every effort of the poor to improve their economic status. To destroy a child because one is unable to afford the costs of his upbringing would be a heinous sin indeed, and abortion for such reasons must be placed in the same category. The life of a poor child can be hard indeed, but many children of poor homes have, by God's grace, overcome their hardships; and who can say that life in poverty is worse than no life at all?

c. A somewhat stronger, or at least more plausible argument is that abortion is sometimes necessary to guard the *psychological health of the mother*. So-called psychiatric indications for abortion are used to justify 30-50 percent of legal abortions—up to 80 percent in ten states with relatively liberal abortion laws. "Psychiatric indications," however, appears to be a catch-all phrase with no clear meaning. Most of those receiving abortions on such grounds are not under the care of a psychiatrist and often have no psychiatrically definable ailment. Further, abortion may very well cause more psychological problems than it eases. Some psychiatrists state that an abortion can lead to more severe mental disturbance, especially if there is some genuine psychological illness present. In general it seems impossible to determine whether an abortion will help or hinder a genuine psychological condition, and many feel that with modern psychological therapies available it makes more medical sense to bring the pregnancy to term in such cases. But what if the situation is complicated by a threat of suicide? Studies show that such threats are not generally carried out and are often manipulative in character. In general, the suicide rate appears to be lower for pregnant women than for other women of childbearing age; the same is true for those who are pregnant out of wedlock. When "psychiatric indications" are weighed against the life of the unborn child, we conclude, the Christian will regard the certain death of the unborn as a greater tragedy than any of the consequences likely to result from rejecting a plea for abortion on such grounds. We would unhesitatingly deny to a mother the right to kill an already-born infant for such reasons; the case for abortion in this context is no stronger than the case for infanticide, and in some respects is even weaker.

d. Some maintain that abortion is sometimes necessary to prevent the birth of *unwanted* children. Evidence indicates, however, that the "wants" of expectant mothers vacillate considerably and offer little indication of whether the child will be truly wanted or appreciated after he is born. Further, a recent California study maintains that 90 percent of "battered" children resulted from *planned* pregnancies—pregnancies that, so far as anyone can tell, were "wanted" when they began. It even appears that since the introduction of the birth control pill, child beating has tripled. This study calls in question the view sometimes expressed that if abortion is made easier (thereby facilitating planned parenthood) all children will be "wanted" and child beatings will decrease. Further, even if a child is in some sense "unwanted" during his childhood, such background need not be an insuperable obstacle to his lifelong—and eternal—happiness. Nor does being "wanted" in childhood guarantee a good life. At any rate, is abortion—death before birth—preferable to an unhappy childhood? We think that this sort of consideration is insufficient to justify abortion. Children who are truly "unwanted" (in a serious sense of that word) at the time of their birth should be put up for adoption. And those concerned about battered children should consider the ugliness of the methods by which unborn children are destroyed in abortions despite their visible struggle for life.

e. What of the use of abortion to protect the *physical* health of the mother (generally called "therapeutic abortion")? Indications for therapeutic abortion vary greatly in their definition: at one hospital one therapeutic abortion per thirty pregnancies was performed, at another, one per 300,000. With such variation, one suspects that other than medical factors enter into some definitions. Yet many doctors maintain that the progress of medical science has made therapeutic abortion generally unnecessary. As long ago as 1951, R. J. Heffernan, M.D., of Tufts University, was quoted as saying, "Anyone who performs a therapeutic abortion is either ignorant of modern medical methods of treating the complications of pregnancy or is unwilling to take time to use them." In this connection it should also be noted that there are certain dangers to the mother in the abortion process itself. Between July 1 and September 4, 1970, out of approximately 19,000 legal abortions performed under a liberalized abortion law, there were eight deaths and ninety-eight instances of complications arising from the operation. The maternal death rate from abortions in Sweden (where again legal abortions are easily obtainable) is thirty-nine per 100,000; in Denmark, forty-one per 100,000; in England thirty per 100,000. These figures from northern Europe are higher than the maternal death rate from all causes in those countries. Abortions performed after the twelfth week of pregnancy are significantly more dangerous. In the light of the rarity of genuine indications for therapeutic abortion and the medical dangers inherent in the operation itself, it seems that there are few if any cases in which abortion might legitimately be recommended on such medical grounds. When we consider further that even in these rare cases the *possible* physical harm to the mother must be weighed against the *certain* death of the fetus, we can conceive of no justification for abortion on such grounds. As for the extremely rare case in which the very *life* of the woman is jeopardized by her pregnancy, we shall discuss that later.

f. An argument with considerable emotional force is the alleged necessity of abortion in cases where pregnancy has resulted from *rape or incest*. Some feel that it is cruel to require a woman to give birth to the child of a rapist. Actually there are extremely few cases of this kind: fewer than one in 5,000 abortions is performed on such grounds, and that figure includes pregnancies arising from statutory rape as well as, we assume, some cases where rape has been falsely alleged. In Washington, *no* documented rape cases resulted in pregnancy over a twenty-year period. But what of the rare cases where such a situation occurs? Until five days after the occurrence of rape, most hospitals will routinely perform a dilation and curettage operation on the woman to prevent any birth arising from the incident. We are unable to endorse this procedure, because it may very well prevent the implantation of a fertilized egg in the womb and thus be in effect the destruction of an unborn child. This result, of course, is most unlikely if the operation is performed within a few hours after intercourse: during that period, the operation is a form of contraception rather than a form of abortion. But in view of the uncertainty of timing, we regard another procedure, an oil douche to prevent fertilization, as preferable from a moral point of view. If, however, neither of these methods is used immediately for some reason and the woman finds out later that she is pregnant, should she seek an abortion? We must reply in the negative. We are here weighing the shame, pain, and inconvenience of the mother against the life of her child, and we have no choice but to decide in favor of the latter. The unborn child must not be put to death for the sin of a parent. A Christian must indeed sympathize with the plight of a woman in such a situation and must be prepared to give counsel, prayer, and other help. In spite of her suffering, she should be helped to see from God's Word what a privilege it is to bring a child into the world and how the child, even from such an origin, may be one of God's elect—a blessing to God's church and to the world. In some cases, it may be best for the child to be put up for adoption, but in any case, his destruction is not the answer.

g. Abortion is also frequently recommended to prevent the birth of *deformed* children. Again, the frequency of such cases is sometimes overestimated. Among pregnancies complicated by rubella or German measles (notorious as a cause of birth defects), only one of four children is born with any deformity, and only 8 percent are born with deformities of a grave character. If a mother's rubella were regarded as adequate ground for abortion, three potentially healthy children would be killed to prevent the birth of each deformed child. From a Christian point of view, such procedures must be rejected decisively. Further: medical science has made great strides recently in diagnosing and treating deformities both before and after birth. We now have access to RH and measles vaccines, and fetal blood transfusions and intrauterine surgery (even heart surgery) are also available. After a child has been born with a deformity, he has access to many forms of therapy; new training techniques for brain-injured and retarded children have been developed. This progress seems likely to continue, but the rate of progress will certainly be slowed if abortion to prevent deformity becomes the general procedure. And a still more important consideration is the following: What man has the right to say that life with a handicap—even a serious handicap—is not worth living? There has never been any evidence that people with birth defects are generally any less happy than other people, or less useful to society, let alone less precious in God's sight. The suicide rate among deformed persons is less than that of the general population. In some cases, handicapped workers have been shown to be more efficient and dependable than the nonhandicapped. Many people have experienced great joy as well as challenge in the rearing of a retarded child. If, however, we insist in spite of these facts that death is better than a deformed life, what will prevent us from applying that principle to those who are born normally, but subsequently become deformed? And what will prevent us from enlarging our definition of "deformity" as a pretext for eliminating all "undesirables" from society? Eugenic euthanasia, infanticide, geronticide—such are the results of the master-race mentality that is only one or two logical steps from the proposal to kill off the deformed before birth. The decisive consideration, however, is that as Christians we must treat the unborn child as a human person, and that human personhood implies a right to life, even when the quality of that life is hampered by deformity.

h. The strongest argument in favor of abortion, however, is that it may sometimes be necessary *to save the life of the mother.* Here it seems to be a question of one life or the other. The sixth commandment requires not only that we refrain from killing, but that we make diligent efforts to preserve life. Thus, it is argued, to allow a mother to die without taking available measures to save her is at least as great a sin as killing an unborn child. The question then becomes whether we kill the child to save the mother, or whether we kill the mother (by our inaction) so as not to do harm to the child. This is indeed a difficult moral question, but (we should again point out) one that arises only with extreme rarity, if at all. As we pointed out earlier (*e*, above), many physicians feel that generally it is far less dangerous today to allow a pregnant woman to deliver her baby at term than to perform an abortion, even in the comparative safety of a hospital. Yet no one is prepared to rule out the possibility that some situation may at some time arise wherein the continued existence of the unborn child is inconsistent with the continued life of the mother. From a Christian point of view, the main problem is somewhat as follows: Granted that the sixth commandment requires us to make diligent efforts to preserve a life, may those diligent efforts include the taking of another life? Surely we would not wish to argue that stealing or committing adultery or false worship are legitimate when done to preserve life in some sense. The situation we are discussing is not strictly analogous to the case of the father who, when his two children fall out of a boat, must abandon one in order to save the other. The father does not *kill* the child he abandons, but simply leaves him in the hands of God, and such is not the case where an abortion is performed to save a mother's life. Nor is the abortion case strictly analogous to a case in which a man, driving with all proper caution, comes unexpectedly upon a group of jaywalkers and finds that he must steer his car so as to hit the fewest number of them. In that case, the driver may kill, but he does not choose to kill; he chooses only to kill some rather than others. But in the abortion situation, an actual *choice to kill* is involved. The abortion case under discussion is more like the situation where a person trying to enter a crowded lifeboat must be killed to prevent him from hindering the survival of the others in the boat. This lifeboat case is, however, almost too close an analogy, for it raises the same problem as the abortion case, rather than helping us to resolve it.

Perhaps the closest *helpful* analogy is the following. A woman walking with her husband in a deserted area is suddenly attacked by an unknown assailant. The assailant is strong, and the husband cannot stop the attack. The husband realizes that merely to wound the assailant may not be sufficient to save the life of his wife, so he picks up a lead pipe, the only available weapon, and delivers a sharp blow to the skull of the attacker. Afterward, he discovers that the assailant had escaped from a mental institution, and thus was, perhaps, of diminished moral responsibility. The husband has intentionally killed a person who could not have been convicted of any crime in order to protect the life of his wife. The moral responsibility of the assailant, or lack of same, was not relevant to his decision. If we are prepared to endorse the husband's action in this situation, on the ground of his God-given responsibility for his wife's safety, then we must be prepared to endorse abortion in cases where the mother's life is jeopardized by pregnancy. Yet even this analogy breaks down at a crucial point, for in the abortion case the husband is under divinely imposed obligation not only to protect his wife, but to protect his child also. Is there reason to suppose that the former responsibility supersedes the latter? Does Exodus 21:15 speak to this issue? At present, we are not prepared to speak to these questions. Some Christians will be able to endorse abortions in such cases with good conscience, and others will not. We are not able at present either to condemn or to endorse the procedure. The question requires further careful study. In general, however, this is the only justification for abortion that we are unable to condemn on Christian grounds.

18. Granted that abortion in nearly all cases must be regarded as murder, does it follow that the Christian should endeavor to protect the unborn child through *legislation*? We answer in the affirmative.

a. We do not, of course, maintain that a fully Christian morality should be legally required of every citizen in our pluralistic society. Regeneration cannot be forced upon people by legal constraint. Protection of the lives of persons, however, has always been regarded as a legitimate function of government both in Scripture and in modern legal systems. In American law this protection is not compromised in the interest of freedom of religion. A Jehovah's Witness who refuses to allow a blood transfusion to preserve the life of his child can be compelled to do so. A Christian who holds that unborn children should be regarded as persons should exert his influence upon legislators (and law-enforcement officials!) to protect the lives of such persons and should not turn away from this task for fear of infringing upon the freedom of religion of others.

b. One objection to strict abortion laws on the above principles is that they discriminate against the poor; for the rich are able to obtain abortions whatever the law, either by traveling to other countries or by paying substantial sums for a competent, though illegal, abortion here. The fallacious premise of this reasoning, however, is that if rich people are able to do something wrong, the law should make it easy for poor people to do it too. This principle would make havoc out of all legal structures. If indeed the law prevents only poor people from doing wrong, then at least it has accomplished *something* worthwhile. In a more profound sense, such a law discriminates against the rich, not the poor, for it fails to protect the children of rich parents and fails adequately to encourage the rich to protect the lives of their children. However, a fair law should indeed be formulated and enforced so as to guard equally against abuse by the poor and by the rich.

c. Some argue also that strict abortion laws are bad because they are difficult to enforce and are not supported by many in our society. The case of Prohibition is sometimes cited as an analogous law in this respect. Such a principle, however, would remove from our books laws opposing racial discrimination, drug addiction, and robberies. Further, granting that Prohibition was as unenforceable as it is often claimed to have been, there is still very little analogy between a law against sipping wine and a law against killing people.

d. It is also argued that strict abortion laws cause people to turn to illegal and often incompetent abortionists and hence result in many deaths that liberalized laws would prevent. Actually it is very difficult to tell how many illegal abortions are performed and how many deaths result from them. Sometimes it is claimed that there are over a million illegal abortions in the United States every year and that 10,000 maternal deaths result from these in the same period. But most advocates of liberalized abortion laws leave quite a bit of leeway in these figures (e.g., "between 200,000 and 1,200,000 abortions")! As for the number of deaths, the figure 10,000 may be grossly inflated. The medical section of the First International Symposium on Abortion (Washington, D.C., 1967) could verify only 235 maternal deaths resulting from abortion in 1965 and felt that a realistic figure including those unreported would be around 500. The U.S. Public Health Service listed only 130 deaths from abortion, in 1968, both legal and illegal. Since only 45,000 women of childbearing age die each year from all causes, it would be incredible to imagine as many as 10,000 dying from any single cause. Of those deaths that have occurred, it is not clear that the illegality of the operations was the major factor. It has been estimated that 70 percent of all illegal abortions are performed by M.D.'s. The inherent dangers of the operation itself (cf. above, section 17, e) seem to be as large a factor in these deaths as is the incompetence of some of those performing it. Furthermore, there is evidence from countries with permissive abortion laws that such liberalization does not put an end to the business of incompetent abortionists. In such countries many women still turn to the unqualified abortionists to save money, to avoid red tape, and to maintain secrecy. It appears that in those countries, as well as ours, more diligent law enforcement, not greater permissiveness, will be needed to put the incompetents out of business.

19. We conclude, therefore, that the Christian should regard the unborn child as a human person made in the image of God. Such a regard for the unborn child will involve rejection of abortion, except possibly in order to save the life of the mother. On the basis of this concern, the Christian should use his influence to promote legislation that will protect unborn human life. Adoption of these general principles, however, does not excuse the Christian from a rigorous self-examination as to the motives of his heart in making decisions in these matters, nor does the adoption of these principles automatically justify any act allegedly performed in accord with them. Further, in counselling with those facing difficult deci-

sions in these matters, the Christian must not use his general principles as a way to avoid wrestling with a particular case. The
agonies of those contemplating abortion must be shared, entered
into, understood, if truly *loving* counsel from the Word of God is to
be given.

BIBLIOGRAPHY

Bahnsen, Greg. *By This Standard*. Tyler, Tex.: Institute for Christian Economics, 1986.

_____. *Lectures on Medical Ethics*. Available on tape from Geneva Ministries, Box 131300, Tyler, TX 75713.

_____. *Theonomy in Christian Ethics*. Phillipsburg, N.J.: Presbyterian and Reformed Publishing Co., 1977, 1984.

Beauchamp, T., and Childress, J. *Principles of Biomedical Ethics*. New York: Oxford University Press, 1979.

Beauchamp, T., and Perlin, S., eds. *Ethical Issues in Death and Dying*. Englewood Cliffs, N.J.: Prentice-Hall, 1978.

Beauchamp, T., and Walters, L., eds. *Contemporary Issues in Bioethics*. Encino, Calif.: Dickenson Publishing Co., 1978.

Bird, Lewis P. "Dilemmas in Biomedical Ethics." In *Horizons of Science*. Edited by Carl F. H. Henry. San Francisco: Harper and Row, 1978.

Byrne, P., and Quay, P., eds. "On Understanding 'Brain Death.'" Omaha: Nebraska Coalition for Life Educational Trust Fund, n.d.

Childress, J. *Priorities in Biomedical Ethics*. Philadelphia: Westminster Press, 1981.

Davis, John J. *Evangelical Ethics*. Phillipsburg, N.J.: Presbyterian and Reformed Publishing Co., 1985.

Feinberg, Joel. *Social Philosophy*. Englewood Cliffs, N.J.: Prentice-Hall, 1973.

Fletcher, Joseph. *Morals and Medicine*. Boston: Beacon Press, 1960.

Frame, J. *Doctrine of the Christian Life*. Unpublished class syllabus.

_____. *Doctrine of the Knowledge of God*. Phillipsburg, N.J.: Presbyterian and Reformed Publishing Co., 1987.

_____. *Report of the Committee to Study the Matter of Abortion*. Philadelphia: Orthodox Presbyterian Church, 1972. I was the chief author of this report on behalf of the committee, which also included Rev. Robert Malarkey and Joseph Memmelaar, M.D. The Rev. Paul Woolley was also on the committee, but he disagreed with the *Report* and submitted a minority opinion. The Report was revised for R. Ganz, ed., *Thou Shalt Not Kill* (New Rochelle, N.Y.: Arlington House, 1978), 43-75.

Geisler, N. *Ethics: Issues and Alternatives*. Grand Rapids: Zondervan Publishing House, 1971.

Harron, F., M. D. Burnside, and T. Beauchamp. *Health and Human Values*. New Haven: Yale University Press, 1984.

Hatfield, C., ed. *The Scientist and Ethical Decision*. Downers Grove, Ill.: Inter-Varsity Press, 1973.

Henry, Carl F. H. *Christian Personal Ethics*. Grand Rapids: Wm. B. Eerdmans Publishing Co., 1957.

_____. ed., *Dictionary of Christian Ethics*. Grand Rapids: Baker Book House, 1973.

Kaiser, W. *Toward Old Testament Ethics*. Grand Rapids: Zondervan Publishing House, 1983.

Koop, C. Everett. *The Right to Live, the Right to Die*. Wheaton, Ill.: Tyndale House, 1976.

Ladd, John, ed. *Ethical Issues Relating to Life and Death*. New York: Oxford University Press, 1979.

Murray, J. *Principles of Conduct*. Grand Rapids: Wm. B. Eerdmans Publishing Co., 1957.

Payne, Franklin. *Biblical/Medical Ethics*. Milford, Mich.: Mott Media, 1985.

Ramsey, Paul. *Ethics at the Edges of Life*. New Haven: Yale University Press, 1978.

_____. *The Patient as Person*. New Haven: Yale University Press, 1970.

Rushdoony, R. J. *The Institutes of Biblical Law*. Phillipsburg, N.J.: Presbyterian and Reformed Publishing Co., 1973.

Schaeffer, F., and Koop, C. Everett. *Whatever Happened to the Human Race?* Westchester, Ill.: Crossway Books, 1983.

Smedes, L. *Mere Morality*. Grand Rapids: Wm. B. Eerdmans Publishing Co., 1983.

Van Til, Cornelius. *Christian-Theistic Ethics*. Unpublished syllabus.

Veatch, R. *Case Studies in Medical Ethics*. Cambridge: Harvard University Press, 1977.

_____. *Death, Dying, and the Biological Revolution*. New Haven: Yale University Press, 1976.

_____. *A Theory of Medical Ethics*. New York: Basic Books, 1981.

INDEX OF SCRIPTURE

127

INDEX OF PROPER NAMES